# tommy'sguidetobeing
# pregnant

By Sarah Levete &
Penny Tassoni

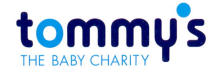

**tommy's**
THE BABY CHARITY

# Help save babies' lives

**Tommy's exists to save babies' lives. We fund pioneering research into miscarriage, premature birth and stillbirth and provide information on pregnancy health.**

Our pregnancy health information service is free of charge, so we are able to provide everyone with the best possible chance of having a healthy pregnancy and a healthy baby. But we need your help.

☐ **Yes, I'd like to make a gift to help Tommy's give every baby the chance to be born healthy**

| Name | Address |
| --- | --- |
| | Postcode |
| Telephone | Email |

☐ **Yes, I'd like to give regularly to Tommy's from my bank account.** Please do not send this form to your bank.

| Bank name | Bank Address |
| --- | --- |
| | Postcode |
| Name(s) of account holder | |

Branch Sort code ☐☐ ☐☐ ☐☐  Bank or Building Society a/c no ☐☐☐☐☐☐☐☐

I would like to give a regular gift of £ ☐ per month/year (delete as appropriate) by Direct Debit 6 5 5 1 3 3

on the 1st/15th (delete as appropriate) of the month, and until further notice (Please ensure the start date is at least one month from today's date)
**Instruction to your Bank or Building Society:** Please pay Tommy's, the baby charity Direct Debits from the account detailed in this instruction subject to the safeguards assured by the Direct Debit Guarantee. I understand that this instruction may remain with Tommy's, the baby charity and, if so, details will be passed electronically to my Bank/Building Society.

☐ **Yes, I'd like to make a single gift**

I enclose a cheque/postal order/CAF voucher made payable to Tommy's, the baby charity

Or please debit my Visa ☐ Mastercard ☐ Switch/Maestro ☐ Amex ☐ CAF card ☐

☐☐☐☐ ☐☐☐☐ ☐☐☐☐ ☐☐☐☐ ☐☐☐

Security code (last 3 digits on your signature strip) ☐☐☐

Start date ☐☐/☐☐ Expiry date ☐☐/☐☐ Issue no (Switch/Maestro only) ☐☐

*giftaid it* ☐ **I'd like my gift to be worth 28% more to Tommy's at no extra cost to me!**

Tommy's can claim back the tax on your gift, increasing its value at no extra cost to you. You need to be a UK taxpayer, paying as much tax as we'd be claiming. If you're not a UK taxpayer, or don't currently pay enough tax, please tick here ☐

| Signature | Date |
| --- | --- |

Tommy's takes data protection very seriously. We promise we will not pass your details to other organisations or charities. If you do not wish to receive further information or appeals from Tommy's about our work, please write to us using our address details listed below.

☐ Please tick this box if you do not wish to receive further mailings from Tommy's.

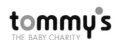

Please return this form to
Tommy's, the baby charity,
FREEPOST LON1053, London EC4B 4BR.

**tommy's** THE BABY CHARITY

TOMMY'S THE BABY CHARITY is a registered charity no 1060508

BP/04

2

# Welcome to the world of pregnancy!

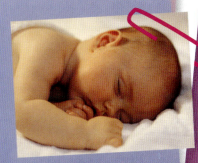

The coming months hold a host of new experiences for you and your family. Whether you planned your pregnancy and have been looking forward to the adventures it will bring, or it was something of a surprise, you are commencing a journey which will bring many changes. Our guide to being pregnant will help you get ready, giving you all you need to know about what's happening to your body and your new baby.

Packed with easy-to-read articles about physical changes, descriptions about who is there to help you and how, and real life stories about others' pregnancies, this guide will answer all your questions and more.

Through all the joys and the challenges your pregnancy brings, we aim to show you the best ways to have a healthy, happy nine months, giving your baby the best possible chance to be born healthy and strong.

Wishing you all the very best for your pregnancy.

From all the team at **Tommy's**

**Remember!** If you have any questions about your pregnancy, you can call our friendly midwives on **0870 777 30 60** who are here to give you all the information you need.

# Contents

**6** — **Welcome to the world of pregnancy**

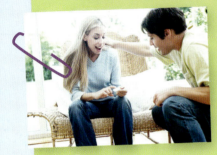

**Weeks 1–12**

Pregnancy is an amazing journey: get prepared and read about your first three months.

**8** — **Time to find out for sure**
Are you pregnant? Time to put that sneaking suspicion to the test

**10** — **Week-by-week guide to your pregnancy, weeks 1–12**
The first weeks – Body changes, emotional upheavals, exercise, and more

**16** — **Morning sickness**
Bucket under the bed – Why? What can I do?

**18** — **Antenatal care – getting started**
Getting good care from the start – how, who and why?

**23** — **Meet midwife, Claire Friars**
Community midwife and health information officer for Tommy's pregnancy health service, Claire tells us about her typical day

**26** — **Know your body**

**28** — **Miscarriage**
Sadly, not every pregnancy goes to plan. We look at the causes of miscarriage and what you should do if you suspect you are having one.

**30** — **Early pregnancy** Your questions answered

**32** — **It's your choice**

**Weeks 13–28**

As your baby grows and your antenatal care continues, you'll be making lots of choices, like what tests to have, and how you want to have your baby. Read on to learn about the next three months.

**38** — **What happens next?**
From now on, your baby will be monitored regularly: learn about the tests on offer and what to expect at your antenatal appointments

**41** — **Meet sonographer, Trish Chudleigh**
Sonographer at a busy London hospital, who scans up to 50 mums-to-be each week, she tells us the joys and challenges that go with the job

**43** — **Antenatal classes**
Your pregnancy care is not complete without your antenatal classes. Join other mums-to-be and learn more about your pregnancy

**46** — **All change – half way there!**
And the growth goes on: what to expect as your body continues to change

**49** — **Where will I have my baby?**

**50** — **Your questions about birth**

**52** — **Mid-pregnancy** Your questions answered

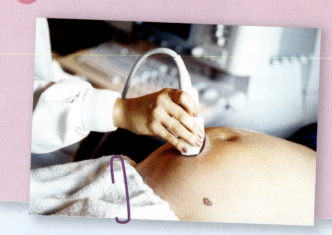

**54** *Not long to go now!*

**Weeks 29–40**
The end is nigh, you're entering your last months. What to expect and how to prepare for your labour.

**57 Meet obstetrician, Dr Louise Kenny**
So what does an obstetrician actually do? Louise tells us about her typical day

**58 Antenatal care – final weeks**
You're being checked more regularly as your body starts preparing for birth

**61 All change – how your body prepares for birth**

**63 Thinking ahead**
Pain relief, birth plans, the kit you'll need – how to prepare as the countdown commences

**This is it – your baby's big day!**

**72** After months of waiting, planning and preparing for your baby, the moment has finally arrived. Read a little about what to expect.

**77 Meet labour ward midwife, Justina**
With up to six women in labour at once, Justina talks us through a typical shift on a labour ward

**78 First minutes of life**
Well done! You may feel totally elated, exhausted, happy, amazed, and probably tired! Time to meet your new baby.

**80 Caesarean section**

**81 Babies who arrive early**

**82 Babies who arrive late**

**83 Birth**
Your questions answered

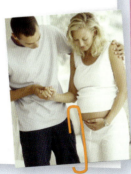

**84** *Happy & healthy*

Your pregnancy affects your life in many ways: from work and pay, to exercise, health and relationships, we look at the big issues.

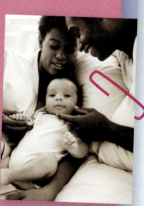

**86 Piling on the pounds**
One woman's story of weight management through pregnancy

**89 Drugs, tablets & pills**
Pregnancy is a time to think about what you're putting into your body. We talk about how drugs can affect your baby.

**90 Time to quit smoking**

**91 Keep fit, keep moving**
Being pregnant is much harder work if you're not taking gentle exercise. Read about the dos and don'ts of pregnancy fitness

**93 Problems in pregnancy**
So many body changes, sometimes it's difficult to tell common niggles from more serious concerns

**96 Feelings & relationships**
Pregnancy can be a testing time – sometimes acknowledging the problems is the biggest step

**98 Count down to fatherhood**
Over to the men! Read about what to expect and how you can be her biggest support

**101 Just like the movies**
Neil tells his story about the birth of his first son

**102 More than one – twins and multiples**

**103 Your rights & benefits**

**105 True or False?**
How much do you know about pregnancy?

**106 Signposts** Useful organisations

**108 Index**

# *Welcome to* *world of*

**P**regnancy is an amazing journey for everyone, especially mum, baby and dad. It's not all easy, but there is a fantastic team of health professionals to support you, and there are many simple things you can do to help you and your baby have a happy, healthy pregnancy.

## How you can tell

Some women feel pregnant even before they know for sure. Others don't have a clue until they do a test to confirm that a baby is on the way. The sooner you find out, the sooner you can start looking after yourself and your growing baby.

*You may be pregnant if:*
- **You've missed a period**
- **You feel more tired than usual**
- **Your bra feels tight**
- **Some foods taste different**
- **You feel sick**
- **You need to wee more often**
- **You feel emotional and tearful**

### My period is late
If your periods are regular, you'll know if your period is late. Then you can take a pregnancy test (see page 8). But if your periods are all over the place, you may not be sure if you have missed one completely.

Missing a period isn't the only sign. If you think there's a chance you may be pregnant, watch out for other clues.

## My breasts feel funny

Some women experience breast tenderness or a tingly feeling in their breasts in the early weeks of pregnancy. Your nipples may look more 'bumpy' than usual or feel heavier. This is all down to the hormonal changes that take place.

## I've got a funny taste in my mouth

Have you suddenly gone off your favourite food or do you have a strange taste in your mouth? These are common signs of early pregnancy.

## I feel so tired

The first few weeks of pregnancy can feel physically and emotionally draining, even though your baby is smaller than a pea. If you do feel tired, and nothing in your life has changed, maybe you are pregnant.

## I need to wee – again!

Do you need to wee more than usual? In early pregnancy, this is because your uterus expands and presses on your bladder and there is an increase in the hormone progesterone.

**Did You Know?** You may have some light bleeding like a light period when you are first pregnant. This happens as the newly implanted egg settles into the uterus. So, if you experience other symptoms and think you could be pregnant, it's a good idea to take a pregnancy test.

# *the*
# *pregnancy!*

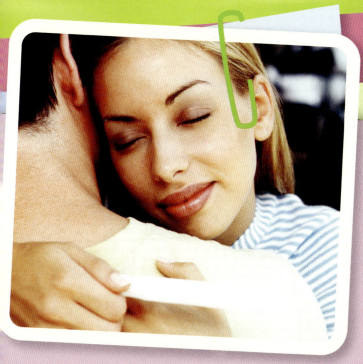

**left** Try and tell
your partner as soon
as you know you are
pregnant. Don't be
worried by his first
reaction – try to give
him some time to let
the news sink in.

## I'm in a lousy mood

It's usual to feel up and down in the
early weeks of pregnancy. So if you feel
emotional and tearful, don't necessarily
put it down to a row with your partner
or a bad day at work.

*Did you know?* Hormones are going
to play a major part
in your life from now
until well after the birth.
These are natural
chemicals in your body that
get your body used to being
pregnant, prepare it for the
birth and then help provide your
baby with milk.

## I feel sick!

Unfortunately, feeling sick can start even before your pregnancy is confirmed. Some
women feel slightly nauseous and others may be actually be sick. And it isn't always
just a morning feeling. It can happen at any time of day (see page 16).

## Top tip

If you travel to work on a crowded bus or train, and need to sit
down, and you don't want to explain that you are pregnant, simply
say you feel faint – someone will give you a seat pretty quickly!

**Check this out** Uterus is
another word for womb. Not sure
what your uterus is or where it
is? Look at page 26 for a basic
biology lesson!

# Time to find out for sure

OK You have a sneaking suspicion … it's time to find out for sure. You can take a test the day after your period was due, to detect a hormone that is released when you're pregnant. This hormone is human chorionic gonadotrophin, or HCG for short. If you are pregnant, there will be traces of HCG in your urine (and blood) from the day after your period was due.

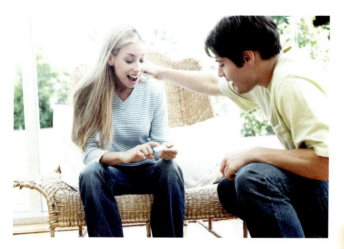

**above** A positive test will set off a whole range of emotions.

**Say again?** HCG is Human chorionic gonadotrophin, the hormone that your body produces when you are first pregnant.

### At the doctor or chemist

You can take a sample of urine in a clean container to the chemist and they will do the test for you, or you can go to the doctor who may offer you a urine test to confirm your pregnancy. Your local family planning clinic or a Brook Advisory Centre (see page 106) can also do a test for you.

### At home

You can buy a pregnancy testing kit from a chemist or a large supermarket and do the test at home. If you do this, follow the instructions carefully. It's best to do the test in the morning before you drink anything – traces of HCG will show more strongly. A strip of chemical on the testing pad or stick changes colour if HCG is present. This means you are pregnant.

If the test is negative, and you still think you may be pregnant, repeat the test a week later.

"It seems obvious now, but it wasn't until I kept feeling sick that I started to click that I might actually be pregnant! It explained why I was so tired and why I hadn't had a period in a while"

**Did you know?** Two weeks after you conceive (when sperm and egg made a match) you are four weeks pregnant! Doctors count your pregnancy from the date of your last period (usually about two weeks before conception).

**Did you know?** Pregnancy lasts an average of 40 weeks (280 days) but only a few babies arrive on their due date. The estimated due date (the day your baby is due) is often shortened to EDD in your notes.

## What to do next

**See your doctor** First, see your doctor who will start to plan antenatal care for you and your baby. Your doctor will look at your medical history to see if you need any special care while you are pregnant – for example, if you have diabetes or epilepsy.

**Talk to someone** Tell your partner as much or as little as you feel OK with. Or confide in a close friend. You may want to chat to your doctor or midwife before telling anyone else. Other sources of help are listed on page 106.

**Take care of yourself** A healthy lifestyle gives your baby the best start in life and there are lots of tips for staying healthy, starting on page 84.

**Chill out** Most women feel a huge range of emotions at this stage. It's natural to find the going tough, so try not to be too hard on yourself.

## Pelvic floor exercises

The pelvic floor muscles are the ones that support all the organs of the pelvis – your bowels, uterus and bladder. Imagine that you are desperate for the loo and are trying to hold everything in. Or that you and your partner are making love and you are squeezing him from inside – that's your pelvic floor muscles at work.

Pregnancy and childbirth aren't kind to your pelvic floor muscles. Hormonal changes loosen them up and the growing baby presses on your bladder. You might find that you leak wee when you cough or laugh, or during exercise. This is called 'stress incontinence'. Then the muscles of the vagina work hard during birth to push the baby out.

It's best to start doing exercises to strengthen your pelvic floor as soon as you can. In fact, you can start right now while you are reading this. Or on the bus, or at work. No one can see you doing them.

As if you were trying to stop yourself weeing, lift the muscles inwards and upwards. Don't forget to breathe! Then let go, and do a few more squeezes. Do this several times a day whenever you remember.

If you find this difficult, your midwife can help you work out whether you're doing it properly.

**Say again?** Antenatal means before birth.

*" I had a sneaking suspicion that I could be pregnant as I was three days late, but my body felt kind of different as well "*

## Q&A

**Q.** When is my baby due?

**A.** You can estimate your due date if you know the date that your last period started. There's a quick way to do this. Say your last period started on 17th October 2004.
**1.** Add a year – 17th October 2005
**2.** Take away three months – 17th July 2005
**3.** Add a week – 24th July 2005. This is just a guess – most babies arrive within a week either side of their due date.

If you don't know when your last period started, or your periods are irregular, the best way to find out your due date is when you have your first scan (see page 41).

**below** You can roughly work out your baby's due date, but most babies arrive within a week either side of this date.

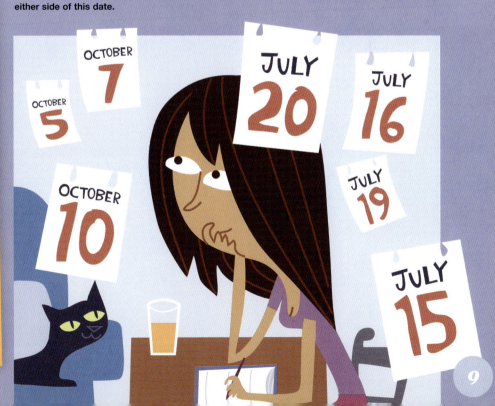

# Week-by-week guide to your pregnancy

## Weeks 1–12

Your pregnancy has three terms, or trimesters. Here, we're looking at the first trimester, which is roughly from week 1 to week 12 of your pregnancy, starting from the date of your last period. This calendar is a guide to what is happening to you and your baby. Don't be alarmed if you don't follow this pattern exactly. Each woman and each baby is different.

**Pregnant freebies!** You can get free prescriptions and dental treatment when you're pregnant. Ask your doctor or midwife for form FW8.

**Say again?** 'Full term' means a pregnancy that lasts between 37 and 40 weeks.

| | Your baby's development | Your body | Healthy tips | Things to do/ that happen | How you may feel |
|---|---|---|---|---|---|
| **weeks 1–5** | Nature has a funny way of working! The early weeks of a baby's development are crucial and the fastest in your baby's growth, but many women don't know they are pregnant for a while. During this time you may feel very tired. You may not know you are pregnant. Don't worry if you've drunk lots of coffee, been to an aerobics class or had too many late nights. Now you know you are pregnant, you can take simple steps to look after yourself and your baby. | | | | |
| **weeks 5–6** | Your baby is just over the size of an orange pip! Her central nervous system, brain and spine are beginning to form. | You may notice some light bleeding or 'spotting'. This is usually caused as the fertilised egg settles in the uterus wall. If this bleeding persists, is heavy or you also have abdominal pain, see a doctor as soon as you can.<br><br>Your breasts may feel heavy and tender. | Start taking folic acid, until week 12. This helps prevent conditions such as spina bifida which affect your baby's nervous system.<br><br>Stop smoking. Cut back on alcohol (see page 88). If you use street or recreational drugs, stop or ask your doctor for advice on stopping safely. | When your pregnancy is confirmed, make an appointment to see your doctor.<br><br>Continue to use condoms unless you are sure your partner does not have a sexually transmitted disease (STD). | Tired and emotional? Don't worry – it doesn't mean you won't be a great mum. It's due to lots of hormones racing around your body. |

| | Your baby's development | Your body | Healthy tips | Things to do/ that happen | How you may feel |
|---|---|---|---|---|---|
| **weeks 6-7** | Your baby is about the length of a kidney bean. Her tiny heart beats and her head is taking shape. Other organs such as kidneys and liver are forming. The neural tube that connects the spine and brain closes. Tiny marks show the developing nostrils and ears. | Your nipples may look darker. This is due to the increase in your blood supply.<br><br>Your body is working harder now and your heart rate increases.<br><br>Hormonal changes may make you feel or be sick – at any time of day.<br><br>Your growing baby is pressing down on your bladder so you may need to wee more often.<br><br>You may feel very tired. | You may be off some foods for a while. Try to keep eating a healthy diet (see page 84). Look at the list on page 87 of foods to avoid. Eat little and often. Try ginger biscuits or rice cakes.<br><br>Keep drinking plenty of water or juice. Avoid fizzy sweet drinks and too much caffeine in coffee or fizzy drinks.<br><br>Check with your chemist before taking any over-the-counter medicines. Some are not suitable for pregnancy. Ask your doctor if it is safe for you to continue taking prescription medicine. Make sure complementary medicines are safe for use in pregnancy. | If you think your job could be a health risk to your pregnancy, tell your employer in confidence about your pregnancy.<br><br>Make an appointment to see your doctor if you have not already done so. He or she fixes up your antenatal care (see page 18).<br><br>You may start thinking about screening tests (see page 40). These check you and your baby for certain conditions. | Your baby is growing at an incredible rate, so rest when you can.<br><br>It can feel like a long wait between telling your doctor and having your first antenatal appointment. You may feel a bit isolated and unsure about the progress of the pregnancy. Ask your doctor if you have concerns about your or your baby's health and chat to a close friend if possible.<br><br>You may feel as if you can't go another 7 months feeling so tired. But it will get better! |
| **weeks 8-10** | Your baby's major organs have started to form. She has tooth buds growing, and you can see her fingers and toes.<br><br>Your baby is starting to move around, but it may be a few weeks before you can feel her kick! | Your waist may be slowly increasing.<br><br>Increased hormones may make your skin a bit spotty.<br><br>Your digestive system is slowing down and can make you feel bloated or give you indigestion and heartburn.<br><br>You may feel a bit dizzy or light-headed. | Keep eating small regular meals. Now is not the time to go on a slimming diet.<br><br>If you use essential oils, check they are ok for pregnancy.<br><br>Keep a supply of energy-rich snacks nearby (such as bananas). | Have a check up with your dentist and tell him or her you are pregnant so you don't have X-rays.<br><br>You may have your 'booking' appoint-ment with your ante-natal team between now and week 14. You may be offered your first scan between weeks 10 and 14. Make a list of ques-tions you want to ask. | You may feel anxious about how you are going to cope or how others will react to the news of your pregnancy.<br><br>Avoid stress wherever possible. If you are fed up and feel tired, take a warm bath, chill to some music, close your eyes and think of your beautiful baby. |
| **weeks 11-12** | Your baby's organs have formed and she can suck, chew and swallow. Her toenails and fingernails are beginning to form. She is beginning to look like a baby, and she's about as long as your little finger. | You may feel warmer and thirstier than usual.<br><br>Headaches are common in the first trimester.<br><br>You may notice a black line called a linea nigra up your belly. This is just darkening skin and will fade after the birth.<br><br>You may begin to look pregnant. | Get plenty of fresh air, and keep up your fluid intake. Try to rest often.<br><br>Wear a good support bra (it's best to be measured in a shop).<br><br>Start practising pelvic floor exercises (see page 9). | Contact your doctor if you have not yet been given a date for your 'booking' appointment.<br><br>Ask your midwife about antenatal or parentcraft classes. They won't take place until mid to late pregnancy, but classes may book up quickly.<br><br>Ask your employer for a 'risk assessment' (see page 48). This helps ensure your work place is safe and comfortable for you and your baby. | You may be feeling quite excited now. The risk of miscarriage declines after 12 weeks and you may want to tell friends and work-mates your news! |

# All change – how your body prepares for pregnancy

This first part of your pregnancy can feel like the hardest. First, there's the amazing news that you are pregnant, which feels exciting for some women and confusing for others. And then there are the huge physical changes that start to happen to your body.

## Common physical problems

Most women have these symptoms in early pregnancy and they are usually nothing to worry about. But if you are worried about any symptoms, or you feel unwell, talk to your doctor or midwife as soon as you can.

| Problem | Why? | Top tips |
|---|---|---|
| **Feeling or being sick** (at any time of the day, not just in the mornings) | Your body is adapting to huge hormonal changes. | If you cannot keep any food down, let your doctor or midwife know. There's lots more about morning sickness on page 16. |
| **Feeling exhausted** | For the first few months, your baby is growing so fast, she is using up a lot of your energy. | • Take some gentle exercise – it can give you more energy!<br>• Rest when you can.<br>• Try to 'book' yourself some time each day, even if it's just ten minutes.<br>• Read a magazine, have a relaxing bath or simply close your eyes for a few minutes and relax.<br>• You may want to tell your employer so she or he will understand why you are not racing around like usual. Ask your employer if you can adjust your working hours while you feel so tired. |
| **Needing to wee a lot** | Your baby is pressing down on your bladder and your kidneys are working overtime to cope with the increase in body fluids. | • Don't cut back on drinking water or juice.<br>• You may want to tell your employer so you have easy access to a loo. |
| **Feeling constipated** | Your digestion slows down when you are pregnant. | • Eat plenty of fruit and vegetables (see page 85).<br>• Take gentle exercise. |
| **Tender breasts** | Your breasts are growing and responding to rapid hormonal changes. | • Make sure you have a well-fitting supportive bra.<br>• Hold a cold damp flannel over your breasts if they feel tender.<br>• Many large department stores offer a bra-fitting service. Take advantage of it – it's free! |
| **Tummy ache** | It's common to feel a little discomfort in your lower abdomen (tummy). | If you also have heavy bleeding or severe pain, see your doctor or midwife as soon as possible. |
| **Headaches** | Rapid rises in pregnancy hormones. | • Take plenty of rest and relaxation when you can.<br>• Drink plenty of water or juice.<br>• Eat small, regular meals.<br>• You can take paracetamol, as long as you stick to the recommended dose. |

| Problem | Why? | Top tips |
|---------|------|----------|
| **Feeling faint** | The extra demand on your body's blood system can make you dizzy. | • Lie down if you can with your legs up.<br>• Breathe slowly and deeply.<br>• Get up slowly.<br>• Take plenty of rest and make sure you can get into the fresh air.<br>• Eat regularly and drink plenty of fluids.<br><br>If you do faint, tell your doctor or midwife as soon as possible. Report any dizzy spells at your next appointment. |
| **Feeling windy** | It's common to feel bloated when you are pregnant, and to fart and burp more than usual. | • Try to eat small regular meals, and avoid gulping them down.<br>• Don't eat too many gassy foods such as beans or fried foods. |
| **Going off sex** | Hormonal changes mean that some women want more sex when they are pregnant. Others go off it dramatically. | • Do what feels right for you. Your baby won't come to any harm when you have sex.<br>• Make sure your partner wears a condom unless you are sure he has no sexually transmitted disease (STD).<br>• Talk to your partner about how you are feeling. |
| **Changing shape** | At the end of this trimester, you may well begin to 'look' pregnant. | • Eat a balanced diet and take some reasonable exercise.<br>• This is not the time to fret about diets and weight gain but it is the time to make sure you have a healthy balanced diet (see page 84).<br>• Unless you suddenly put on excessive weight or lose too much, you will probably only be weighed once at your booking appointments. |

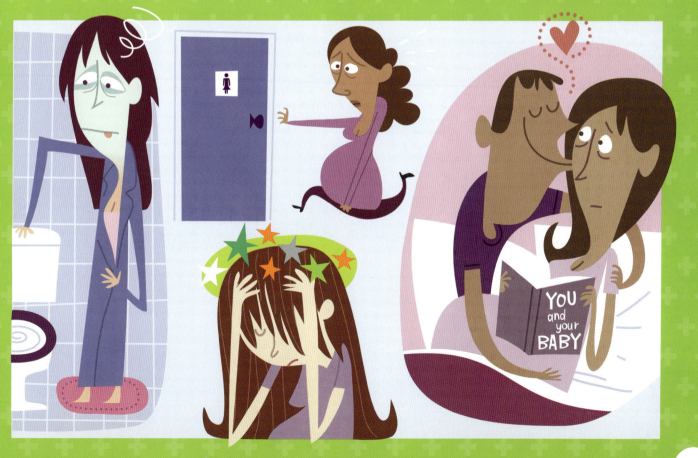

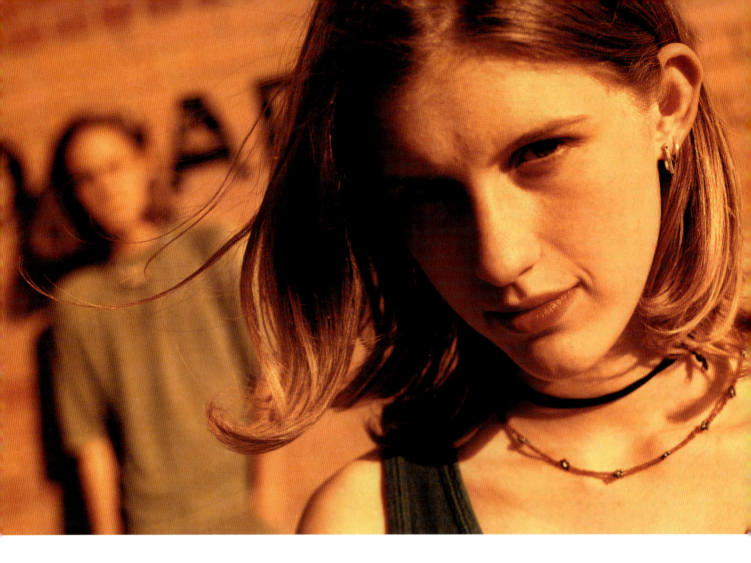

## Feelings about being pregnant

Many women feel anxious, moody or fearful in early pregnancy and even if someone says 'Don't worry' – you probably will!

| Problem | Why? | Top tips |
|---|---|---|
| **Feeling low** | There's a lot going on and your body is still changing rapidly. Hormones are playing havoc, and it's understandable if you feel weepy. | Just because you're not jumping up and down for joy doesn't mean you're not going to be a great mum. It's natural to have mixed feelings. If the feelings are overwhelming and don't go away, tell your doctor or midwife how you feel. |
| **Fear of miscarriage** | If you have previously lost a baby, you may understand-ably feel very anxious. | Ask for reassurance from your healthcare team and make time to relax. Make extra sure that you eat well and rest as much as you can. |
| **Worry about a previous abortion** | Some women are nervous about their pregnancy because they feel uncomfortable talking about a previous abortion. | Your healthcare team are not there to judge you but to help you have a healthy, happy pregnancy. Your midwife doesn't have to record your previous abortion in your hand-held notes where friends or family may see, but they do need to know, so it is really important to be honest! |

Try to find some time each day to close your eyes and imagine holding your beautiful new baby. Feels good, doesn't it?

## Introducing exercise

Unless you have a special care pregnancy or an existing medical condition, pregnancy is not an excuse to be a couch potato! In fact, exercise will help with many irritating pregnancy problems, such as constipation, difficulty sleeping and even feeling tired. If you do exercise classes, go for low-impact exercise rather than activities where you are jumping or running on the spot. Try swimming, or yoga – make sure you tell your exercise teacher that you are pregnant. If you can hold a conversation normally while exercising, and don't feel too out of breath, then the exercise you are doing is probably all right.

### Top tip

When you first see your doctor about your pregnancy, ask him or her if your current or planned exercise routine is OK for you and your baby.

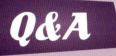

# Q&A

**Q.** I'm really into clubbing. Do I have to give all that up now?

**A.** Being pregnant doesn't stop you having fun – but you need to be aware of your body's and your growing baby's needs. If you go clubbing, avoid getting overtired, and make sure you drink plenty of water and avoid smoky atmospheres. The smoke from someone else's cigarettes can get into your baby's developing lungs and damage them. Don't use recreational or street drugs – they can be incredibly harmful to your baby and remember to limit the amount of alcohol you drink (see page 88).

**Q.** Should I start exercising?

**A.** Yes, but don't start a major exercise routine if you haven't done very much till now. Avoid contact sports such as karate or rugby where you could crash into another person. Avoid hard games of tennis or squash that could put too much strain on your tummy. Exercise will keep you feeling good (see page 92 for ideas).

**Q.** I really wanted a baby but now I'm pregnant everything seems to be going wrong. My boyfriend doesn't want to know and I'm worried how I'll cope on my own. It's not how it's meant to be.

**A.** The most important thing now is to look after yourself and your growing baby. You've been longing to have a baby. Your boyfriend may just need time to take in the news of your pregnancy. If he can't support you emotionally, let your friends and family support you, or talk to your doctor or midwife.

**Check this out** There's more about exercise and posture on page 91.

**right** Good posture will help make your pregnancy more comfortable.

**Q.** I'm so pleased to be pregnant. I've been trying for ages. But now I feel so tired and weepy. I don't have the energy to enjoy this.

**A.** The exhaustion does pass. These first few months are tiring because your baby is developing so fast and is using energy from you. Make sure you are eating well (see page 84) and take time for plenty of rest. Even if you are working hard and home doesn't seem that restful, there are ways to make time for you.

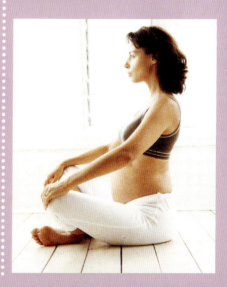

# Morning sickness

**N**ausea and sickness are common symptoms in early pregnancy and nearly half of all pregnant women will have some sign of them.

## Top tips for morning sickness

Different things work for different women. You might not be able to completely stop your sickness or nausea, but some of these things can help. Something you try this week may not work the next, so be ready to try new remedies.

### In the morning ...

- Try to raise your blood sugar before you get up by eating a biscuit or a piece of chocolate with a drink of water
- Eat slowly and sip slowly
- Get up as slowly as you can
- Avoid sudden movements

### At other times ...

- Try to have small healthy snacks every 2–3 hours
- Keep sipping water or other drinks
- Avoid alcohol and fatty foods
- Lie down and rest, even for a few minutes, during the day
- Work out which foods and smells make you worse and try to avoid them

### Foods to try

- Foods and drinks with ginger in them, such as ginger biscuits, chamomile and ginger tea, ginger ale
- Crystallised ginger
- Sparkling water
- Fruit and herbal teas (but not raspberry leaf tea)
- Ice cubes
- Milk
- Pasta, bread or water biscuits

### See your doctor if ...

- You cannot keep any food or drink down at all
- You have lost weight
- Your vomit contains blood or is dark
- Your urine is very dark in colour or there is very little of it
- You feel dizzy
- If you are worried or do not feel that you can cope

## Q&A

**Q. Why do I feel so awful?**

**A.** Your body is reacting to higher levels of the pregnancy hormone HCG (see page 8). Symptoms are often at their worst when you first wake up, which is why it is called morning sickness. This is partly because you haven't eaten and your blood sugar is low. Some experts believe that morning sickness is the body's way of insisting that you rest as this seems to be the one thing that can really make a difference.

**Q. How long will this go on for?**

**A.** For most women, the first 12 weeks are the worst and you will gradually feel better. By around 14 weeks, you will probably find that the sickness has completely gone away.

**Q. How will my baby grow if I'm not eating normally?**

**A.** You only need to worry if you are being so sick that you cannot keep down any food or water. Try and eat 'little and often' rather than big meals. Choose healthy snacks such as sandwiches and fruit rather than crisps. Try to drink a small glass of water every hour you are awake. And keep taking folic acid for the first 12 weeks.

### Top tip

Some women find acupressure wristbands helpful. These are also used for travel sickness and you can find them in the travel section of your chemists.

# Bucket under the bed

**F**eeling sick all the time can come as a shock when you don't know much about being pregnant. Jackie tells how she survived morning sickness and counted the days till it was over.

I got pregnant really quickly and knew within the first week of missing my period. I realise, looking back, that I didn't know much about pregnancy at all! I had no sisters or friends with babies, so while I wanted a baby, suddenly finding that I felt sick all the time came as a big shock.

I had vaguely heard of morning sickness, but had no idea that you could feel and be sick at any time – day, afternoon, evening and night! Mine started during the sixth week and I felt wretched. I needed a bucket under the bed, as in the morning for the first hour, every movement I made would make me sick.

## Resting

I was given all kinds of advice and I did try the cup of tea and the biscuit in the morning, but although it helped a little, it didn't make a huge difference. The only thing that helped was resting and I did find that if I could take my time getting up, it was much better. I also found that eating small snacks throughout the day was better for me.

I also became really sensitive to smells. The smells of soap, fruit, smoke and petrol would make me instantly sick, which meant that I couldn't go out much in case I got a waft of them. I got fed up of hearing that morning sickness only lasts for the first twelve weeks. When you have still another five weeks to go, it seems like forever. It was true for me though.

## Well enough to Hoover!

By about the twelfth week, I felt much better and then one Saturday, it just lifted. My partner came back from work and found me up and even doing a bit of Hoovering! Before that, I hadn't had the energy to do anything like that. I was also ravenous for the first time and I had a meal and kept it down. It was wonderful. After that, the rest of my pregnancy went smoothly, and even the birth was a doddle. The only thing that I wish I had known was that feeling sick can be a sign of a strong pregnancy. In the worst moments, I had thought that if anything had happened to the baby, I would not try again.

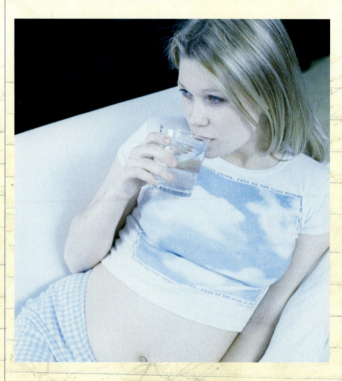

**above** Try to drink a small glass of water every hour you are awake.

*"The rest of my pregnancy went smoothly, and even the birth was a breeze "*

# Antenatal care – getting started

Antenatal care means care while you are pregnant. It is care of you and your growing baby. Your antenatal care team are specialists. Ask them all the questions you want. They are there to reassure you, check your health, to spot any possible problems and to offer you and your baby any special treatment if you need it.

## Top tip

Check that your doctor's surgery has your current address and phone number. If you move, tell your doctor and midwife.

**Don't forget** If you have any concerns between your antenatal appointments, speak to your doctor or midwife. You can also talk to a midwife by phoning Tommy's pregnancy information line on 0870 777 30 60. Don't worry in silence!

## Doctor first

The first thing to do is see your doctor. She or he is unlikely to do another pregnancy test but will ask you the date of your last period. Don't panic if you don't have a clue. Your first scan (see page 41) will help to show when your baby's due.

The doctor will arrange for your antenatal care to start, so this is the time to discuss what you want and what is available.

If you have any health concerns at this stage, tell your doctor. If you are worried about how conditions at work may affect your baby's health, discuss it with your doctor. If your job presents significant risks to your healthy pregnancy, the doctor can fill in a form called a MED 3. Your employer must act on this.

## If your home pregnancy test is positive...

1. Make an appointment to see your doctor. You can discuss which type of antenatal care is available to you and which you would prefer.

2. You can make a huge difference to your baby's growing body and your health during pregnancy. Check out the tips on page 84.

3. Your doctor will arrange your first 'booking' appointment with your antenatal care team.

4. You'll have regular follow-up appointments, depending on your health and pregnancy.

## Top tip

If you don't speak or understand English very well, tell your GP at your booking visit who may be able to arrange for an interpreter to be at your booking appointment. Or you could ask an English-speaking friend or family member to come with you to interpret. Remember they'll be asking personal questions so think about whether you'll want them to know.

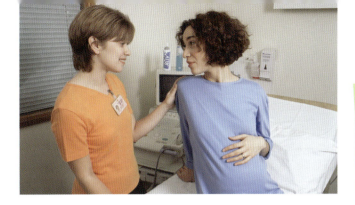

**above** Your doctor can reassure you and look out for possible problems.

## Top ten tips – what you can do for you and your baby

1. Attend your antenatal appointments
2. Eat a healthy diet
3. Drink plenty of water
4. Stop smoking
5. Cut back on the alcohol you drink
6. Stop using recreational or street drugs (ask your doctor first if you are addicted to them)
7. Start taking folic acid (until week 12 of your pregnancy)
8. Take some regular exercise
9. De-stress
10. Phone a friend if you feel fed up

## Where do I go for antenatal care?

*You may be offered your antenatal care*
**at your local hospital**
**at your doctor's surgery**
**at your doctor's surgery with the community midwives**
**at home with visits from the doctor or midwife. This depends on your health and the care available in your area.**

## Top tip

When choosing antenatal care, think about how easy it will be to get to your appointments.

## Q&A

**Q.** Will I always see the same person at my antenatal appointments?

**A.** Under the team or domino scheme, you will see a midwife from one group or team. (Remember though, midwives have holidays and sick leave like the rest of us, so sometimes you may see one of their colleagues).

**Q.** Will my antenatal appointments be at the hospital, the doctor's or a health centre?

**A.** Care may be shared between your doctor and the hospital.

Discuss with your GP what happens in your area.

**Q.** Can I still go to hospital antenatal classes if I choose a home birth?

**A.** Yes, just make sure you tell your midwife you would like to book for antenatal classes.

**Q.** Can the midwife I see for my antenatal appointments deliver my baby?

**A.** This may be possible if the domino or team midwifery scheme is available in your area.

### Types of care
- Your care may be **shared** by your doctor and a hospital.
- Some areas have a **domino** scheme. This means you see a midwife from a team operating in your area and one of the team goes to hospital with you when you are in labour or will be with you at home if you have a home birth.
- Some areas have **team midwifery**. This means you see a midwife from the team at each visit and during your labour.

### Finding the care you want

If your doctor doesn't offer the care you want, you may be able to register with another doctor for care of your pregnancy, and still see your own doctor for all other health matters. It's worth thinking about how easy it will be to get to another doctor, especially if you work or have small children. Your local health authority can give you a list of doctors who have a special interest in pregnancy and childbirth.

# Your booking visit

Your first appointment is called the 'booking' appointment. This is the big one and it happens when you are around eight to twelve weeks pregnant. Be prepared to spend at least an hour at this first appointment. Don't worry, following ones won't be so long, but there is usually a lot of waiting. If you have other young children, take along plenty of games and snacks to keep them amused. Don't forget snacks, magazines or books for yourself.

## What happens at booking?

First, your midwife will ask you lots of questions and write down the answers. This is called 'taking a history' and is the most important part of your booking visit. These questions may be about:

- your medical history
- any medication you are taking for an existing condition (such as diabetes, asthma or epilepsy)
- your family's health
- your partner's family's health and medical history (he may like to come to answer these questions)
- how much you smoke
- how much alcohol you drink
- your sexual health
- your relationship with the father-to-be
- your ethnic origin and that of the father
- previous pregnancies
- your health since you've been pregnant
- whether you have any religious requirements

**Check this out** Don't understand your notes? Check out the jargon buster on page 24.

## Why all the questions?

Your antenatal team are there to look after you and your growing baby. The answers to all the questions help your antenatal team be aware of any particular risks to you and your baby. For example, some ethnic groups are more at risk of some medical conditions than others, so it helps the team to know mum and dad's ethnic origin. Ask if you want to know why a particular question is relevant.

## Be honest!

Whatever you say to your midwife or doctor is in confidence (they can't tell your family or friends your details, but do tell them if there is something you especially want kept private). They will not judge you. They only want to build up a picture of your physical and emotional health so you can have a happy, healthy pregnancy. If you suffer from an eating disorder, have mental health problems or are about to be thrown out of your flat, tell your midwife, who may be able to put you in contact with useful support organisations.

## Don't panic!

If you have lost contact with your baby's father or know little about his medical history, don't worry. Any details you can give your midwife will be useful. If you don't know the answer to a question and are able to find out later, keep a

*Things you may want to discuss at your booking visit:*
- **where you can give birth**
- **health queries**
- **worries about your lifestyle before you realised you were pregnant**

note of the question and let your antenatal team know the answer at the next appointment.

## What else happens?

### Height and weight

You'll be measured and probably weighed, although in many cases this is the only time you will be weighed.

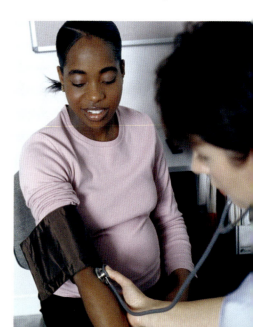

## Blood pressure checks

The reading from this first blood pressure check will give your antenatal team a measure on which to judge future blood pressure checks which are done at each appointment. High blood pressure needs to be monitored for the safety of you and your baby.

## Urine (wee) sample

You will be asked to give a sample of wee to check for traces of protein, which could be a sign of a urine infection which is common in pregnancy; or sugar, which could be a sign that you're developing diabetes in pregnancy. The midwife or nurse will give you a container for this.

## Blood sample

At this first appointment, you will be asked to give a blood sample. This includes information about your blood group and can also show if you have syphilis, hepatitis B, HIV, sickle-cell or thalassaemia, or suffer from anaemia (lack of iron) or if you have been vaccinated against rubella (German measles). If you have any worries about this blood test, chat to your midwife.

## Ultrasound scans

Most women have a first scan of their baby around week 12 of the pregnancy. Earlier scans may be offered if your doctor feels there may be a medical reason to do so.

## Cervical smear test

If you have not recently had a smear test, you might be offered an appointment for one. It does not affect your baby, but helps identify any women at risk of cervical cancer.

**left** Blood pressure checks are an important part of your antenatal care.

### Top tip

The Maternity Alliance has easy-to-read fact sheets on rights for pregnant women. See page 106 for details.

**Check this out** See page 39 for details about different routine and diagnostic tests you may be offered.

## Tests

Your midwife or doctor will explain any tests available to you (see page 39) and what the results mean for you and your baby. It's up to you whether you have these tests. Take your time before deciding, and ask your midwife or doctor as many questions as you need.

## Work and money

Your midwife or doctor will be able to tell you about the different benefits available to you. She or he will also ask you about your work, to make sure it is safe for your pregnancy. If you don't already have one, ask for your free prescription form.

### Notes...

During your booking appointment, midwives fill in a record. These are your notes and you will usually be given them to look after. Take good care of them, as there is no copy! Keep them handy in case of an emergency. Feel free to read your notes and ask if you don't understand anything.

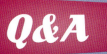

### Q&A

**Q.** Will I have an internal examination?

**A.** No, it's most unlikely you will have an internal examination at this early stage. You will have one when you go into labour to find out how far advanced your labour is. Your doctor or midwife calls this a 'vaginal' examination or VE.

**Q.** I don't want to have a blood test. Can they make me?

**A.** No, but a blood test gives your antenatal team important information about your health that may affect the care you and your baby later need. If you are frightened of any of the tests, tell your midwife.

**Q.** Do I have to take my baby's dad with me?

**A.** No. Do what feels comfortable for you. Perhaps you want someone with you in the waiting area, but say if you would prefer to see your midwife in private.

**What's a scan?** An ultrasound scan uses high-pitched sound waves to create a picture of your baby's development.

# Meet the team

Your antenatal team is a group of different specialists who all work together. You may wonder who all the different people are, especially if they do not wear white coats or uniforms.

## Doctor

Your doctor or GP (general practitioner) is your family doctor. He or she will arrange your antenatal care and look after your general health. In between your antenatal appointments, you can always make an appointment to see your doctor about general health queries or pregnancy queries.

## Midwife

The midwife is a health professional who specialises in looking after pregnant women, delivering their babies and caring for them in the first days after birth. Midwives work in hospitals, doctors' surgeries and in the community, visiting women at home. Your midwife may be male or female. Some midwives work mainly in hospitals. Others, called community midwives, work mainly in doctors' surgeries or seeing women at home. If you have a home birth, a community midwife will be present and support you during the birth.

Some women will see the same community midwife when they go to the doctor's surgery, for antenatal check-ups, but different ones when they go to the hospital. It is also possible to pay for an independent midwife. Contact the Independent Midwives Association for further information (see page 106 for contact details).

## Students

It's common in hospitals and in the community to be seen by a student midwife who is working and observing alongside a qualified midwife. You can say if you would prefer the student not to be present.

## Obstetrician

Your obstetrician is the hospital doctor or consultant who specialises in pregnancy and birth. She or he works in a hospital and heads a team of registrars and senior house doctors, midwives and nurses. You will probably only see your obstetrician if you have a special care pregnancy or if you need extra help to deliver your baby (see page 76). However, in some hospitals the obstetrician may see you even if your pregnancy is straightforward. If you have concerns about your pregnancy, you can always ask to see an obstetrician.

You may meet ultrasound technicians called sonographers or radiographers who scan you and read the results. You may also meet a physiotherapist specially trained to support pregnant women and new mums. He or she will advise you about getting back into shape after the birth.

## Health visitor

Your health visitor may visit you in your home before the birth but will definitely visit you about 10 days after the birth. She or he will make sure you and your baby are in good health, and offer support and information until your baby goes to school. They carry out the checks and immunisations to ensure your baby is developing properly.

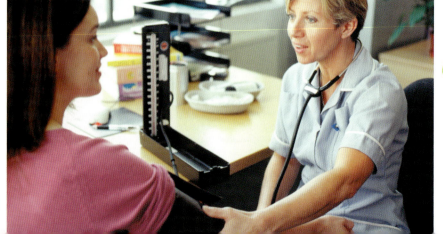

**Did you know?** The care your friend or sister had in another area may not be on offer to you, because the type of antenatal care you receive depends on where you live. But wherever you are, your antenatal team will do everything they can to make you feel as comfortable as possible.

**left** Your antenatal team are there to help, ask them anything you need to know.

# A midwife's day

Claire Friars (25) is a community midwife in South East London. She also works on the pregnancy information helpline for Tommy's, the baby charity.

I usually get up at around 7am and am definitely not a morning person! Fortunately, my partner Ade is not that sociable in the morning either. I have a light breakfast, but catch up again on food when I get to work at about nine o'clock.

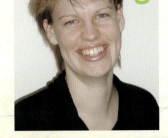

My working day usually begins with a team meeting when we allocate visits. I particularly like these visits as I get to meet people in their own homes and I can check on mum and baby and answer their questions from the first few days of having the baby at home. Getting to the visits is not always as relaxed, especially if the traffic is bad!

## Visits

The reasons for my visits can vary, although we always try and prioritise the first visits for the most urgent cases. Last week, for example, my first visit was a postnatal visit to see a mum whose premature baby wasn't feeding very well, to see how things were going. It took a while, but we were able to get the baby breastfeeding and the mum felt more confident.

Visits to mums are really useful as they give women a chance to ask questions in private without other people around. Some people worry about what their homes or even what they look like, but I can honestly say that we are not into checking the state of their living rooms nor the state of their nightwear. We're just there to support women in pregnancy and straight after birth.

Once the morning visits are over, I grab a quick bite to eat and catch up with my colleagues. A couple of times a week, I then go on to to run an antenatal clinic for one of the local doctors. These clinics are an essential part of looking after women as regular check-ups can make all the difference in a pregnancy. It also gives us time to meet and get to know women if we see them regularly.

## Pregnancy information line

Three days a week, I switch roles and travel to Tommy's, the baby charity's office in central London. I start by answering e-mail queries that have come in during the morning and then take my turn answering the phone queries. The pregnancy information line (0870 777 30 60) is very popular and we get lots of questions each day, although no two days are ever the same.

*There is no time limit and women can phone in as often as they like.*

It's not just women – some men also phone in to get help which is really nice because it shows that they feel it's their responsibility too.

While some calls last just a few minutes, others can last a lot longer, especially where a woman is feeling anxious or has had an experience that she really needs to talk through. There is no time limit and women can phone in as often as they like. Occasionally, women phone us back to let us know how they are doing. One lady who had had a miscarriage and was naturally worried about her next pregnancy, phoned us back the other day to let us know that her baby had arrived safely. It was really satisfying to hear that her pregnancy was a success and that we'd been able to help.

The afternoon goes really quickly and there is a great team spirit in the office. In this kind of work that is important, because sadly pregnancy is not always plain sailing and some calls are about problems in pregnancy.

*These visits are really useful, as regular check-ups can make all the difference in a pregnancy*

# What do my notes mean?

**W**hen the midwife hands you your notes, you'll want to see what's going on. But what does it all mean? Don't worry. Here's our guide to the abbreviations and terms. And if there is something you don't understand, ask.

| Abbreviation | Definition |
| --- | --- |
| BP | Blood pressure. This measures the force with which your heart pumps blood around the body. Two numbers are given, such as 120/70. Your antenatal team check your blood pressure regularly and note a rise in the lower figure, which can show high blood pressure. This can be a sign of problems such as pre-eclampsia (see page 58). |
| Cx | Cervix – the neck of the uterus, which stays closed while you are pregnant and then opens (dilates) when you go into labour (see page 26). |
| EDD | Estimated due date – the day your baby is due (see page 9). |
| Fe | Fe is the chemical symbol for iron. |
| FH | Fetal heart – your baby's heartbeat. The word fetal means 'of the baby'. |
| FHHR | Fetal heart heard regular – this means the midwife or doctor heard your baby's heart. |
| FMF | Fetal movement felt – this means the midwife or doctor felt the baby move. |
| Hb | Haemoglobin – the part of red blood cells that carries oxygen round the body and needs iron. |

**right** Ask your midwife if you find your notes confusing.

### Top tip

Keep your notes in a safe place, and tell your partner or a close friend where they are, just in case. Your notes are an important part of your antenatal care, and can be read and understood by any hospital or antenatal care team.

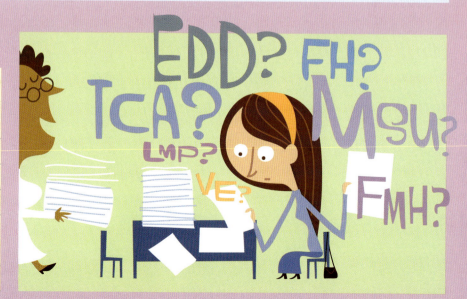

| Abbreviation | Definition |
| --- | --- |
| **Height fundus** | The fundus is the top of the uterus (or womb). As your baby gets bigger, so the uterus will become larger and higher. This is what gives you the bump! Midwives and doctors measure how high the fundus has reached. This will be written down in centimetres. |
| **LMP** | Last menstrual period. |
| **MSU** | Midstream sample of urine. |
| **NAD** | Nothing abnormal detected. |
| **Oed** | Oedema (swelling) – which whilst often normal, can be a sign of a serious condition called pre-eclampsia, so your midwife and doctor will keep an eye on any swelling. |
| **Para 0** | Woman has no previous pregnancy that has gone beyond 24 weeks. |
| **Para 1** | Woman has one child or a pregnancy that went beyond 24 weeks (2 for 2 children, and so on) |
| **PET** | Pre-eclamptic toxaemia (pre-eclampsia, a potentially dangerous condition). |
| **Primigravida** | A woman who is pregnant for the first time. |
| **Multigravida** | A woman who has been pregnant before – may include previous miscarraige. |
| **TCA** | To come again – if your midwife or doctor wants to see you for another appointment to monitor your condition. |
| **TRACE** | This means that a tiny amount of substances like sugar or protein has been found in your urine. If more than just a trace is found '+' will be used. |
| **VE** | Vaginal examination. |

Later in your pregnancy, your midwife and doctor will write some other terms in your notes that describe how your baby is lying.

## Top tip

If you don't understand what your midwife or doctor is saying, ask them to explain it in a different way so you do understand. They won't think you are silly.

**Check this out** Until week 8, health professionals call your baby an embryo. After this it is called a fetus, which means little one!

**Did you know?** Your midwife may put your notes in a coloured folder. Sometimes first-time mums-to-be may have a different colour folder from second-time mums.

# Know your body

OK, admit it! Did you fall asleep in your biology lessons at school? Do you know where your cervix is? Many women don't. You may feel more comfortable if you know which part of your body your midwife is talking about and where it's supposed to be. Read on and find out more.

## Your body

**Areola** The coloured part around the nipple that often darkens in pregnancy.

**Breasts** While you are pregnant – and for a while afterwards – your breasts will dramatically change in size and appearance. Don't worry, it's nature's way of providing instant food for your baby.

**Nipple** The nipple is the part that juts out, although some people use the word to describe the whole area.

**Diaphragm** This is the muscle at the base of your chest that helps you breathe. As your baby grows, your diaphragm gets a bit squashed. This can make you feel a little breathless.

**Veins** During pregnancy, the veins, which supply blood to the breasts, are more apparent.

**Stomach**

**Liver**

**Intestines**

**Kidneys**

**Uterus**

**Fetus** This is roughly how big your baby is at 12 weeks. Your womb will be slightly larger than usual and may push on your bladder a little.

**Cervix**

**Rectum** The last part of your large intestine before it meets the outside at the anus.

**Bladder** Your urine (wee) is stored in your bladder. Increased pressure on the bladder can make you want to wee more, especially in early and late pregnancy.

**Vagina**

## Close up inside

**Ovaries** You have two ovaries, one on each side, where your eggs are stored. After you conceive (when an egg and sperm meet), you will not release any more eggs until well after the birth of your baby.

**Fallopian tubes**

*Did You know?*
There is a huge variation in the size and shape and colour of women's genitals (sexual organs)

**Cervix** Your cervix is the opening to the uterus. It's at the top of the vagina and during pregnancy is closed by a plug of mucus. The cervix opens or dilates when you give birth to allow the baby through your vagina.

**Pelvis** Your pelvis is a basin-shaped structure that supports your spinal column and hip bones

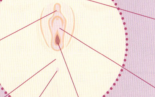

**Uterus** Before you become pregnant, your uterus (also called your womb) is the size of a pear. This is where your baby will live and grow. The top of the uterus is called the fundus (see page 25).

**Vagina** The passage that leads from the outside to the cervix and uterus. Also called the birth canal, during labour it stretches to allow the baby through (and returns to its regular size afterwards!)

## Close up outside

**Pubic hair** This grows over the pubic bone area and on the outer labia.

**Clitoris** A part of the vulva that is responsive to stimulation.

**Vulva** The term used to describe the clitoris, the opening of the vagina, the labia and the opening to the urethra.

**Perineum** This is the area between the vagina and the anus. This area becomes more elastic during labour to allow the baby through the vagina.

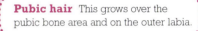

**Vagina opening**

**Anus** Where the rectum meets the surface and bowel movements pass through.

*Did You know?*
Your uterus starts off as the size of a pear, weighing about 40g (1½ oz). By the end of a nine-month pregnancy, it weighs about 800g (28oz). It will have grown to an incredible 38–40cm (7½–8 inches) and can hold about 5 litres (9 pints) of liquid.

## Your baby at weeks 37–40

Later in pregnancy, your internal organs are moved aside to make room for your baby to grow. This is what causes many of the symptoms you feel in pregnancy like heartburn, feeling windy and constipation.

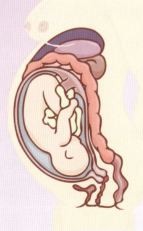

# Miscarriage

Unfortunately, some pregnancies will end early. This is something that many women dread, especially if they have already had a miscarriage before or have known someone who has. We look at the causes of miscarriage and what you should do if you suspect that you are having one.

## Q&A

**Q.** How common are miscarriages?

**A.** Miscarriages are more common than you might think. It is thought that up to one in five pregnancies will naturally come to an early end. This might sound scary, but many miscarriages occur before women even realise that they are pregnant, especially if they have an irregular cycle. The only thing they might notice is that their cycle is longer and that the bleeding is heavier.

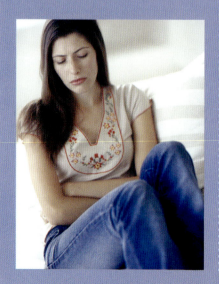

**Q.** When do miscarriages happen?

**A.** Most miscarriages are 'early' and happen within the first 12 weeks. This is the time when the cells are dividing and forming the baby. A 'late' miscarriage is one that happens between 12 and 24 weeks and is much less common.

**below left** Miscarriages are more common than you might think.

### Ectopic pregnancies

Some pregnancies fail because the fertilised egg does not settle in the correct place. Instead of bedding down in the side of the uterus, some stay in the fallopian tube (see page 27). In many cases, the pregnancy then ends naturally, but in some cases the fertilised egg continues to grow. As there is not enough room in the fallopian tube, this becomes very painful and, if left untreated, will cause serious problems, so the pregnancy has to be terminated – the baby cannot continue growing here.

If you have had a positive pregnancy test and have sharp, strong abdominal pain in your stomach area, you must get immediate medical help.

**Q.** What causes a miscarriage?

**A.** There are many causes of miscarriage, although at least half are thought to be genetic – at the moment of conception, some genetic information may be missing or damaged. This means that the early development of the baby cannot continue, so the pregnancy ends naturally. Other common causes include the failure of the fertilised egg to embed itself into the uterus, and cases where the mother has a virus such as rubella or chicken pox.

**Q.** Will it happen again?

**A.** Most women who have a miscarriage will go on to have a perfectly healthy pregnancy and baby later on. But that doesn't stop them worrying, and they may find it very hard to relax in their next pregnancy. The Miscarriage Association (address on page 106) offers support and information for women who have miscarried.

A very small number of women have a medical problem that makes their bodies end the pregnancy early.

**Q.** What should I do if I think I am having a miscarriage?

**A.** Severe abdominal pain, with or without bleeding, can be a sign of miscarriage, although some women may realise without any pain or bleeding that they no longer feel pregnant. If this happens to you, you must phone your doctor or midwife straight away. If this is not possible, go to the accident and emergency department at your local hospital. If you are bleeding, put on a sanitary towel or fold up some tissue. Don't use a tampon.

**Q.** Does bleeding always end with a miscarriage?

**A.** No. Some women have 'breakthrough' bleeding at the time in the month when their period would have been due. The baby is fine.

*Always seek medical help if …*
- **You experience any strong abdominal pains**
- **You begin to bleed, even lightly**
- **Your baby's movements have reduced or stopped**
- **Your waters have broken**

**Q.** What might happen next?

**A.** You may be offered a scan to confirm you have experienced a miscarriage. If you are still bleeding, you're likely to be kept in hospital until the bleeding has stopped. If you're not bleeding you may require a small operation, called an ERPC (which stands for evacuation of retained products of conception). You will be given an anaesthetic during this procedure, which clears your womb.

# My midwife was brilliant

Kylie thought her miscarriage was a punishment for having an abortion when she was 16 – her midwife helped to put her mind at rest.

We had been together for a couple of years and we wanted to start our family. I fell pregnant really quickly, which was great and we were just so excited. I couldn't believe our luck. I told my mum and my sister straight away and I even went out and bought a few little bits, although at the back of my mind there was a little voice saying that it was all too good to be true.

About four weeks after I found out I was pregnant, I woke up with a kind of dull period pain that just got more cramp-like. Later on at work, I went to the loo and saw that there was some blood. I just froze. I didn't know what to do. It sounds silly but my first thought was to try to put a tampon in or something to stop the bleeding. I told my boss that I had to get home.

## Scan

I called Mike, but only got his voice mail. I then got my mum. She picked me up from work in a taxi and we went straight to the hospital. At the hospital, they were really kind and lovely. They took me down for a scan to see what was happening. The scan showed that nothing had really grown and that the pregnancy had ended a couple of weeks before.

All I could think of was that I had been punished because when I was 16, I had had an abortion. When I started to cry, the midwife was brilliant and when I told her about the abortion, she was really nice. She told me that this wouldn't have been why the baby didn't grow and that it wasn't my fault.

Mike came up to the hospital to collect me afterwards and he was really nice about it. To be honest, it took me quite a few months to get over it and I would often find myself crying over things especially at the time when the baby would have been due.

*At the hospital, they were really kind and lovely*

## Pregnant again

About a year later, I fell pregnant again. I was really nervous and the first weeks seemed to crawl on day by day. Getting to past the tenth week felt like a relief, but it wasn't until I was about 20 weeks that I really felt that it would not happen again. Now I have Gracie, I can look back and feel a bit more positive, but it was really hard going at the time.

# Early pregnancy – your questions answered

## Q&A

**Q.** What does a positive pregnancy test mean?

**A.** A positive result definitely means you are pregnant. A negative result shows you are not pregnant.

**Q.** Does my doctor repeat the test?

**A.** Because home pregnancy kits are very accurate, your doctor will not usually repeat a test.

**Q.** Is the test always correct?

**A.** 98% of pregnancy tests are accurate. If a test shows a negative result, but another test a week later shows positive, this is because you release more HCG in the first 12 weeks and the first test may not have picked it up.

### Top tip

Don't want to tell the girls at work you are pregnant but you think that not drinking alcohol is a giveaway? Just say you have an upset tum.

If you still think you are pregnant even though a couple of tests show negative, it's a good idea to check with your doctor.

**Q.** My friend saw the same midwife all the time. Can I do that?

**A.** This depends on where you live. In some places it may be possible to see the same midwife each time. The midwife may also attend your birth at home or be with you at the hospital. This is called the domino or team system and if you want to see the same midwife, ask your doctor about it.

**below** Your midwife is there to put your mind at rest about any worries you have.

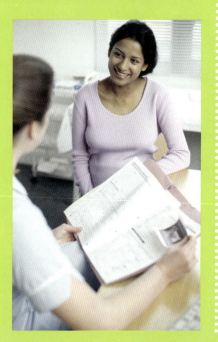

**Q.** They'll think I'm going to be a terrible mother because I was taking drugs when I was pregnant.

**A.** No-one will judge you. They simply need to know as much as possible about you and your baby so they can ensure you have the best care and the best chance of a happy, healthy pregnancy and birth.

**Q.** I've had an abortion before but my partner doesn't know.

**A.** Ask to see your midwife alone (perhaps tell your boyfriend you feel embarrassed in front of him). Or take the phone number of the hospital or health centre and phone your midwife to arrange to speak to her privately.

**Q.** I can't spare the time to go.

**A.** A couple of hours does seem like ages to be at one appointment, especially if you have a demanding job or young family as well. But antenatal appointments keep an important check on you and your baby and can pick up any problems at an early stage.

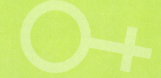

**Q.** My employer won't give me the time off to go.

**A.** Your employer is breaking the law if she or he doesn't give you the time to go to your antenatal appointments (but if you are an agency worker, you may not be paid for time off). If you have any queries, contact the Maternity Alliance (see page 106). It's a good idea to give your employer as much notice as possible about when your appointments are.

**Q.** Is there anything I can do to prevent a miscarriage?

**A.** No-one can guarantee a pregnancy, but a healthy diet and lifestyle (see page 84) will give your baby the best possible start.

**Q.** It sounds silly, but although we have been trying for over a year, I just don't feel happy.

**A.** We cannot always control our emotions and it's normal to react to a new pregnancy differently from the way you'd imagined. Now that you are pregnant, try to relax and be yourself.

**Q.** When can I tell everyone the news?

**A.** You choose. You might be so excited that you want to tell everyone straight away. Or you might want to wait until you know that all is well. Try to tell at least one close female friend, maybe someone who's had a baby herself and knows how you feel.

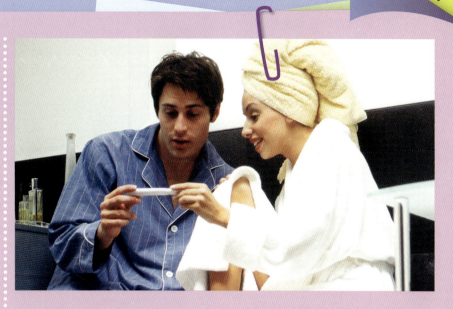

**above** Your partner may be delighted that you are expecting his baby – or it may be a shock for him. Give him time.

**Q.** Help! This wasn't planned and I am very worried about telling my partner.

**A.** First, you need to get your own thoughts in order, especially if you are worried about what your partner will say. It may help you to confide in a close friend or talk to a nurse at your family planning clinic or doctor's surgery. Most women agree that it's best not to put off the moment and to tell your partner early on. His first reaction may not reflect what he really feels – like you, he will be in shock. Try to give him some time to let the news sink in.

**Q.** What do I tell my partner?

**A.** Tell your partner as much or as little as you feel OK with at this stage. If you feel unsure about the pregnancy, you may want to discuss it with your partner or a close friend. Or you may want to chat to your doctor or midwife before telling anyone else.

### Pregnant on the pill?
If you became pregnant while you were on the pill, stop taking it as soon as you are sure you are pregnant. If you became pregnant while using the contraceptive intrauterine device (IUD), tell your doctor or midwife as soon as possible. They can advise you if the IUD should be taken out or if it is best left in place.

### Top tip
Do you have a cat? If so, make sure you wear gloves if you touch cat poo. If it gets in you mouth or bloodstream, it can cause an illness called toxoplasmosis, which can seriously harm your baby. Wear gloves if you garden in soil where cats may have pooed!

If you have a question that isn't answered here, call Tommy's pregnancy information line on **0870 777 30 60** and speak to one of our experienced midwives.

31

# It's your

As your antenatal care gets under way, you'll be making lots of choices – such as what tests to have and where and how you want to have your baby. And you'll have more questions to ask. This section guides you through this next three months.

## Weeks 13–28

In the second three months or 'trimester' of your pregnancy, you may really start to feel that you are pregnant. With luck, you will also feel well – which will come as a great relief if you have been struggling with sickness and tiredness. Watch how your body changes over the next few weeks. You will gradually see your 'bump' emerging and later start to feel your baby moving. This is a time of fast growth for your baby. Many women find this the easiest part of the pregnancy.

As well as routine tests and scans, you may be asked if you want additional tests. The decisions that you will make will be very personal – for example, do you want to know if your baby is a boy or a girl?

You will also start thinking about where and how you would like to have your baby. While this will partly depend on where you live and on your medical history, there are still plenty of choices for you to make. If this all seems a little scary, don't worry. Your midwife will be there to support you and tell you what your choices are. You'll go from novice to expert in just a few weeks!

Opposite is a guide for this part of the pregnancy. You might find that exact timings for antenatal care appointments are different in your area. This calendar is only a guide to what is happening to you and your baby. Don't worry if things don't exactly follow this pattern.

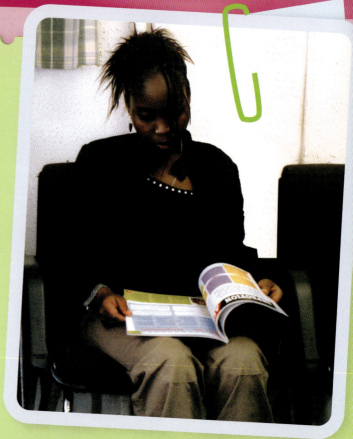

**above** Reading and finding out more about pregnancy and birth helps you make choices about where and how you have your baby.

# choice!

weeks 13-15

| Your baby's development | Your body | Healthy tips | Things to do/ that happen | How you may feel |
|---|---|---|---|---|
| The placenta is your baby's life support system, supplying oxygen and nutrients. The placenta takes over from your ovaries, producing hormones to keep the pregnancy healthy.<br><br>Your baby has her very own unique set of fingerprints!<br><br>Your midwife may be able to hear your baby's heartbeat. | Morning sickness may well have disappeared.<br><br>You may feel fluttering-like movements, but many women don't feel their baby move until around 23 weeks. | You don't need to 'eat for two' but you do need to eat food that is good for you and your baby (see page 84).<br><br>Drink plenty of water (eight glasses a day if possible!) | Give your employer a letter saying you are pregnant. It's important to put this in writing. To qualify for maternity pay and benefits you must let your employer know by week 25. Your employer must make sure your workplace is free from risks to your pregnancy, and make other arrangements for you if necessary.<br><br>Check out what maternity leave and/or pay you are entitled to. (see page 103).<br><br>Read about the tests and scans that you might be offered (see page 39). | Many women feel relieved to be past week 12, and feel they have more energy. Enjoy the next few months. |

| | Your baby's development | Your body | Healthy tips | Things to do/ that happen | How you may feel |
|---|---|---|---|---|---|
| **weeks 16–17** | Your baby's ears are beginning to develop. She will be getting used to the sound of your voice and the beat of your heart.<br><br>The baby is covered in fine hair called lanugo. | You may begin to notice that your waistline has begun to disappear.<br><br>You may have a stuffy nose or suffer from nosebleeds.<br>Your gums may bleed a little.<br><br>This is due to those hormones again! | See your dentist if you have not already done so. | You may have your second antenatal appointment now. Appointments may be monthly from now. You may have a blood test to see if your baby is at risk of conditions such as spina bifida and Down's syndrome.<br><br>If you choose an amniocentesis (see page 39), this will be done around this time. | You may feel relieved that you have got this far, but worried about the next stages and the choices you have to make.<br><br>Try and take some time out to talk about your feelings with your partner or a good friend. |
| **weeks 18–20** | This is a busy time for your baby's growth. Your baby lays down fat under his skin for warmth and energy.<br><br>Your baby has been practising breathing movements, in and out. He is getting very active now and may even move in response to noise!<br><br>He can hear sounds. | You may feel the baby now elbow or kick you!<br><br>You may notice dark spots on pale skin and white patches on dark skin. These disappear a few months after the birth.<br><br>Stretch marks are common in pregnancy, and there's little you can do to avoid them, but you can take care of your skin to reduce the effects.<br><br>Your breasts may start to leak colostrum, your baby's first milk.<br><br>You may notice that you sweat more than before. | Keep up with those pelvic floor exercises (see page 9). They will make a big difference after the birth.<br><br>You may need to check the fitting for your bra. | You will usually have another ultrasound scan (see page 41) between weeks 18 and 23.<br><br>Your midwife will give you form MATB1 around this time. It confirms your estimated due date. You will need to give this form to your employer so you can claim leave and pay due to you (see page 103). | You may feel a bit clumsy and forgetful – it's natural in pregnancy – those hormones again! |
| **weeks 21–22** | Halfway there! Your baby is growing hair and her teeth and gums are forming. | You may notice an increase in vaginal discharge. If it is smelly, itchy, or a yellowy greenish colour, contact your doctor or midwife. You may have an infection that needs to be treated.<br><br>You'll probably feel your baby move soon.<br><br>If you are lucky, a glowing skin may replace spots!<br><br>You may suffer from piles. | Do not use a tampon. Use a pad if the discharge is heavy.<br><br>Make sure your diet is rich in calcium, which is good for you and your baby's bones. Calcium is found in foods such as dairy products and broccoli. | You must let your employer know in writing that you are pregnant and when you want to start your maternity leave by week 25 of your pregnancy. | Reality check time. You are going to be a parent. It'll soon be harder to take time off on your own. |

| | Your baby's development | Your body | Healthy tips | Things to do/ that happen | How you may feel |
|---|---|---|---|---|---|
| **weeks 23–25** | Your baby can cough, hiccup and even suck her thumb! | You may crave certain foods.<br><br>You may have back-ache (see page 46).<br><br>You may notice some slight swelling in your feet and ankles (see page 47).<br><br>Your legs may cramp. (see page 37). | You'll put weight on quickly now.<br><br>Eat healthy foods – too many fatty and sugary foods will make you put on more weight than you need to.<br><br>If it's summer, make sure you drink plenty of water, and stay out of the midday sun.<br><br>Your body temperature is higher when you are pregnant, so it's easy to overheat.<br><br>If it's winter, wear plenty of layers that keep you warm but that you can peel off if you feel hot. | Have fun patting your tummy and talking to your baby. Encourage your partner to do so as well. | Bigger. You may feel that you are moving differently. And other people may start to notice. |
| **weeks 26–28** | If your baby was able to stretch out fully, she could be 37cm (14ins) long!<br><br>Her eyelids open and she can even respond to light outside the uterus.<br><br>Your baby has periods of sleep and has periods of activity! See below for more on baby movement. | You may feel constipated (see page 47).<br><br>A hormone called relaxin softens your ligaments. It's easy to pull a muscle, so go easy. | Eating fibre-rich foods and drinking lots of water will help prevent constipation and piles. | Around this time, you may have a blood test to check for anaemia (lack of iron). Iron is essential for your baby's development. | You may be quite forgetful. Keep essentials like keys, purse or mobile by the front door so there's no mad rush when you go out. Ask your partner to put them there if he finds them somewhere else! |

*Seek medical help if you:*
- **have sharp abdominal pain**
- **are bleeding (even a light spot)**
- **have a vaginal discharge that smells unpleasant or is green, brown or red**
- **feel that you are leaking fluid which is not urine**
- **notice that your fingers or legs have swollen**
- **have persistent headaches**
- **have blurred vision.**

*Did you know?* If you are carrying twins or more, you may experience some of these pregnancy symptoms earlier than other women.

**below** Can you and your partner or a friend take a short break? Travel becomes more difficult after week 30, and many airlines won't let women travel if they are more than 32 weeks pregnant. Wherever you go, take your hospital notes!

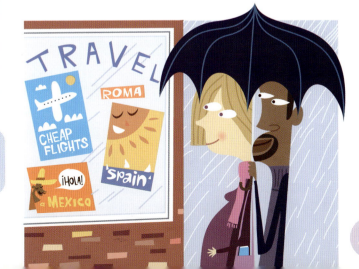

Some mums feel their baby move from as early as week 14. Others don't feel anything until after week 22. Your baby will have periods of great activity and then periods of rest.

**Say again?** Nutrients are the substances in food that provide your body with essential vitamins and minerals. You'll find more about healthy eating starting on page 84.

Your baby's eye colour appears around week 31. But her real eye colour won't appear until six to nine months after birth!

## Q&A

**Q.** My baby doesn't seem very active. What shall I do?

**A.** If after the 28th week of pregnancy, you don't feel your baby move for ten times in a day (from the time you wake up to the time you go to bed), see your doctor or midwife as soon as possible or go to the hospital to check everything is OK. They will monitor the heartbeat of your baby. If you are worried about this before 28 weeks, see your doctor or midwife, or go to the hospital if they are unavailable. If you'd like to focus on your baby's movements, you may like to start a 'kick chart'

If you are thinking about dyeing your hair, stop a moment. Your hair may come out a different colour from the one you expect – pregnancy hormones can make your hair react in strange ways! And your skin is more sensitive so it's a good idea, if you are used to a dye, to have a patch test.

**right** Ooh, was that a kick? Your baby's movements start as tiny fluttering feelings.

### Fact File

**Placenta** The placenta is your baby's life support system, inside the uterus. It supplies nutrients and oxygen from you to your baby. It passes your baby's waste back to your body for you to dispose of. The placenta also produces essential pregnancy hormones.

**Amniotic fluid** Your baby is cushioned from bumps by a protective liquid bubble, called amniotic fluid. When your 'waters break' (see page 73), the amniotic fluid gushes or trickles out of your vagina. This means you are about to go into labour. If your waters break you must go to hospital immediately. Without amniotic fluid, your baby is no longer protected and is at risk of infection.

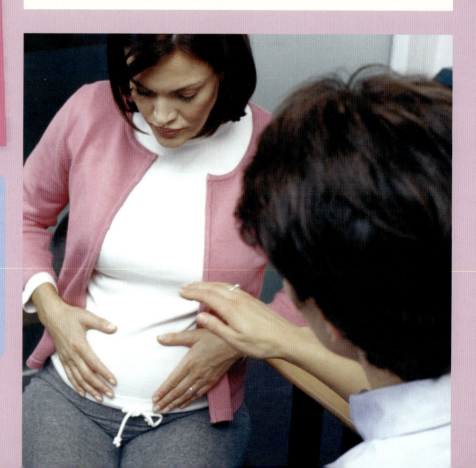

## Fact File

**Hormones – horrid but helpful!** You've heard a lot about them, but what exactly do they do, apart from make you tearful and moody?

| Hormone | What it does |
| --- | --- |
| Human Chorionic Gonadotrophin (HCG) | Stops your periods while you are pregnant. A high level of HCG will give a positive pregnancy test. |
| Human Placental Lactogen (HPL) | This helps the production of milk (and in doing so, makes your boobs bigger!) |
| Relaxin | This hormone softens your ligaments and prepares your pelvis to stretch to allow your baby through. Although you can stretch more, you can also pull a muscle more easily. |
| Oestrogen | Responsible for many things in pregnancy including developing milk glands in your breasts and causing the uterus to grow. |
| Progesterone | Stops your monthly period. It relaxes muscles and joints to prepare your body for labour and your baby's growth. But it can also cause constipation and backache! |
| Melanocyte Stimulating Hormone (MSH) | This can darken parts of paler skin in pregnancy. |

### *Top tip*

You may get cramp, a sharp knot of pain in your leg or foot. You can help avoid it by drinking plenty of water and taking some exercise. It may help to take calcium supplements or drink more milk.

If the cramps are very frequent or if there is a sore swelling on your leg that feels hot to the touch, seek medical help immediately – this could be a sign of a deep vein thrombosis.

**Say again?** A deep vein thrombosis is a blood clot that blocks a vein, usually in the leg. If the clot loosens it can work its way to the lungs and can cause death. Pregnant women are more at risk because hormonal changes make the blood clot more easily. Keeping mobile, drinking lots of water and wearing support stockings can all prevent DVT.

*Did you know?* Many of the ingredients of your own diet will pass across the placenta to your baby's bloodstream – so think carefully about what you eat.

*Did you know?* From the moment sperm and egg meet and match, your baby's genetic map is already in place. This means that you and the dad have equally contributed to your baby's looks and physical being, inside and out.

# What happens next?

From now on, you and your baby will be monitored regularly. Your antenatal appointments are a two-way communication. Your doctor and midwife can keep a check on your health and your baby's development using a series of tests and scans. The appointments are your chance to ask lots of questions about these tests. This information will help you decide what to do next.

## Timescale
### After your booking appointment at around 12 weeks, it is likely that you will have antenatal appointments at around:

**16 weeks** Receive the results of any tests you have had (see page 39).

**18-23 weeks** Ultrasound scan at the hospital as well as your regular midwife appointment.

**26 weeks** Check the size of your abdomen.

**28 weeks** Check the size of your abdomen. You will also be offered a test for anaemia.

At each antenatal visit, your midwife will test your urine and take your blood pressure. Each woman is different, and treatment is tailored to the needs of you and your baby, so don't worry if you and a friend have appointments at different intervals.

**right** Ask your midwife if you don't understand what the test results mean for you and your baby.

## Top tip

If you can't make it to one of your antenatal appointments, let the hospital or your midwife know. If you miss an antenatal appointment, make another one. Each appointment is important. Routine blood pressure checks and urine tests can pick up early signs of infection even if you feel fine. These infections need to be treated for the health of you and your baby.

## Tummy checks

Your midwife feels your tummy to work out the position of your baby and the height of your uterus. This is called palpation. It helps to work out the size of your baby. As a rule of thumb, for each week of pregnancy your uterus grows one centimetre. Once she knows the position of your baby, your midwife will also listen for his heartbeat at each appointment.

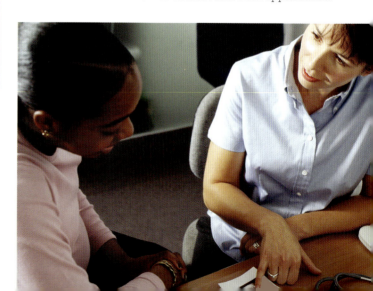

## To test or not to test

You may be offered all sorts of tests while you are pregnant. It's important to understand why you are being offered each test, what the risks are, and what the test will tell you about your pregnancy. This information may help you to decide whether you want to take the test. Some conditions in a baby may not be detected by any antenatal test, even scans.

## What to expect

Before you have any test, your midwife or doctor will explain what the test is for. Your midwife or doctor will explain that it's your choice whether you have the test – if you don't want it, you say so. They will tell you the results of the test and what that means for you and your pregnancy.

### Routine (screening) tests

Routine tests are offered to most pregnant women. These tests identify and support the small number of women who may be affected. The results of these routine tests will not tell you for sure if your baby has a particular condition, but show if you are a higher risk and if you need further diagnostic tests. You'll find a chart of routine tests – and what they identify – on page 40.

## Other tests

### Triple test

A blood test called a triple test screening includes AFP (Alpha-fetoprotein screening), and works out whether your baby is at risk from Down's syndrome and other conditions. It is done between weeks 16 and 20. This test is not always right – sometimes it will show the baby is likely to have it but then further tests show up as negative. If the risk is high, you may decide to have a diagnostic test such as amniocentesis.

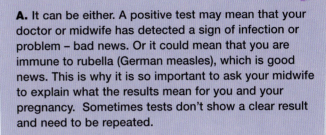

**Q.** Is 'positive' good or bad news?

**A.** It can be either. A positive test may mean that your doctor or midwife has detected a sign of infection or problem – bad news. Or it could mean that you are immune to rubella (German measles), which is good news. This is why it is so important to ask your midwife to explain what the results mean for you and your pregnancy. Sometimes tests don't show a clear result and need to be repeated.

### Nuchal translucency scan

The nuchal fold is a little scrunch of skin at the back of the neck. Everyone has one, but babies with Down's syndrome have been found to have a larger nuchal fold. The nuchal translucency scan helps your antenatal team to work out how likely it is that your baby has Down's syndrome or some other condition.

## Diagnostic tests

If your routine tests are OK, then you may not need a diagnostic test. Diagnostic tests are only offered to women whose routine tests have shown a higher risk of genetic or structural disorders. Some of the most common diagnostic tests include chorionic villus sampling and amniocentesis. These both use needles to take samples from your belly, and so carry a small risk of miscarriage.

### Chorionic villus sampling (CVS)

Done between weeks 10 and 13, chorionic villus sampling can tell you if your baby has Down's syndrome or other conditions such as sickle-cell disease and thalassaemia. Using a thin needle and guided by ultrasound, the doctor takes a sample from the placenta. The test carries a 1% chance of miscarriage – that means 1 in 100 women may have a miscarriage after a CVS.

### Amniocentesis

Done between weeks 16 and 20, amniocentesis can diagnose Down's syndrome and other conditions. A thin needle is inserted into your abdomen and a sample of the amniotic fluid surrounding the baby is taken. One woman in 100 may have a miscarriage after an amniocentesis.

Waiting for the results of amniocentesis or the CVS can be stressful, as they can take a week or so.

### Fact File **Think about it**

Before deciding to have a diagnostic test, consider:
- how the results could affect your feelings about the pregnancy
- the risks to your baby from the tests

Some women choose to have tests if they're in a high-risk group (like women over 35) or if a routine test shows a high risk to their baby and they feel strongly that either they'd terminate the pregnancy if their baby had a serious condition, or they need time to prepare for having a special needs baby.

## Routine tests

| Tests for | How and when | Why |
|---|---|---|
| **Blood pressure** | Measured with a blood pressure cuff at every appointment | Raised blood pressure can be a warning sign of pre-eclampsia (see page 58). |
| **Bacterial infection without symptoms** | Urine sample, done at booking appointment or later | Treatment can prevent an early birth. |
| **Hepatitis B virus, a liver infection that is potentially serious for mother and baby** | Blood test, done at booking appointment or later | Vaccination of the baby at birth can prevent it from contracting the condition and developing debilitating conditions resulting from a failure of liver function. |
| **Human immunodeficiency virus (HIV) that can lead to auto-immune deficiency syndrome (AIDS)** | Blood test, done at booking appointment or later | Treatment during pregnancy can reduce risk to baby. |
| **German measles (rubella)** | Blood test checks if you are immune (have either had it before or have previously been vaccinated against it), done at booking appointment or later | Can cause blindness, deafness, heart problems and other development problems in the baby, so if the test shows you are not immune, you will be advised to avoid contact with people who are likely to have the condition, including young children. You will also be vaccinated after you have given birth to protect you and baby in any further pregnancies. |
| **Syphilis, a sexually transmitted disease** | Blood test, done at booking appointment or later | Mum and baby can be treated with antibiotics during pregnancy. If left untreated it can lead to premature birth, miscarriage or disability. |
| **Full blood count (also checks for anaemia, a lack of iron)** | Blood test, done at booking appointment and then around 28-32 weeks | You can be given iron supplements. |
| **Blood group** | Blood test, done at booking appointment or later | If you are rhesus negative you could have problems in future pregnancies – but these can be prevented with 'anti-D' injections. |
| **Protein** | Urine sample, done at every antenatal check | Raised levels can be a warning sign of infection or pre-eclampsia (see page 58). |
| **Sickle-cell and thalassaemia** | Blood test, done at booking appointment or later<br>*NB: most women will be offered this test* | Rare conditions, both lead to a form of anaemia, which can cause damage to major organs and susceptibility to infection. If your baby is at risk you and your partner will be offered further tests. |
| **Chromosomal defects** | Triple test or nuchal translucency scan (see page 39) | Chromosomal defects include conditions such as Down's syndrome, which means your baby will have special needs unique to that condition. If your baby is at risk you will be offered further tests. |
| **Structural defects** | Triple test or nuchal translucency scan (see page 39) | Structural defects include conditions such as spina bifida, which means your baby will have special needs unique to that condition. If your baby is at risk, you will be offered further tests. |

**Other tests** Blood tests may be offered if you are at high risk of carrying sickle-cell disease and thalassaemia. These are inherited blood disorders that affect some ethnic groups more than others.

## Ultrasound scans

Different hospital trusts offer scans at different times, so don't worry if your antenatal care doesn't exactly fit the timescale below. It often depends on which hospital you attend, and how your pregnancy is progressing.

### 10–14 weeks

*The first scan:*
- **confirms the estimated due date (by looking at the baby's size)**
- **checks if there is one or more babies!**
- **may be used with a nuchal scan to assess the risk of Down's syndrome or other conditions.**

### 18–23 weeks

*The second scan shows:*
- **how your baby is growing**
- **the health and position of your placenta**
- **if there are any visible problems (anomalies)**

## What happens during a scan?

You lie on the examining table and a sonographer spreads a cold sticky gel over your tummy. He or she rolls a small scanning device across your tummy. This sends pictures of what's going on in your uterus to a computer screen. These pictures can be printed.

## Relax!

Lying down with your belly exposed can be scary. Breathe deeply, and tell the sonographer if you feel very nervous.

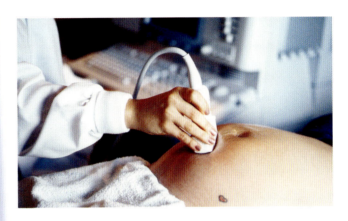

**above** Ultrasound is like a window into your baby's world.

## Honesty is best

Trish Chudleigh is a sonographer, teacher and researcher in a busy London hospital. She scans around 50 women a week.

My department runs three clinics each morning, and two each afternoon. As well as doing around 50 scans a week, I teach and research. I keep up to date because the technology is constantly changing.

I try to make sure that the women I see at the end of the day get the same quality of service as those at the start. I also aim to keep to time so that women are not kept waiting. Each scan usually lasts around 20 minutes. I produce images of the fetus, take measurements and interpret what they mean. I check that the baby is developing well.

The skilful and sometimes hard part of my work is explaining the results. I have a professional duty to be honest, and while most of the scans show healthy babies, occasionally they reveal unexpected things. As I talk through the scan, I try to gauge the reactions of women and their partners, so I can prepare them for news that I think will come as a shock. Twins are a good example of this, triplets even more so!

Occasionally, I have to tell parents that their baby has a medical condition or has died. We talk through what might happen next. Parents naturally find being given bad news difficult but most prefer to be dealt with honestly. When couples return with the next pregnancy, they remember me, and they know that when I say the baby is fine that I mean it.

Parents often ask us about the sex of their baby — we have a look, but a lot depends a lot on the position of the baby. It's lovely for women to come with their partners, family, or close friends. It means that they can feel a part of the pregnancy at an exciting time.

# Two women – two choices

**T**wo mothers tell two different stories of the choices they made in pregnancy, and how they were happy and supported in their choices.

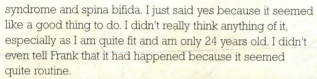

## Yes, I wanted the amnio test

### Kayleigh 24, with baby Emily, 3 months

I was offered a blood test at 15 weeks to detect Down's syndrome and spina bifida. I just said yes because it seemed like a good thing to do. I didn't really think anything of it, especially as I am quite fit and am only 24 years old. I didn't even tell Frank that it had happened because it seemed quite routine.

I was at home when the phone rang and the hospital said that they had made an appointment for me to come in the next day. I was really shocked because I had just assumed that I would be fine. We went along and the consultant explained that the test had showed that I had a 1 in 75 chance of having a baby with Down's syndrome. Frank and I just looked at each other. The consultant said that it was possible to check if the baby had Down's syndrome, but that this would mean having an amniocentesis. The consultant was really good and explained what this would mean and that it did carry a small risk of miscarriage. She also suggested that we went home and thought it over before making a decision. That night we spent a long time talking about it. Frank was brilliant and said that in the end it had to be my decision as I was the one carrying the baby. I decided that I would prefer to know one way or another. We didn't decide what we would do if the test came back and showed there was a problem. Just making the one decision about whether or not to have the amnio was hard enough!

The amnio was arranged for later that week and Frank came with me. I felt confident when they did the amnio. I could see where the needle was and where the baby was. Afterwards, I just knew that it would be fine. Waiting for the result felt like forever. Your belly is getting bigger and you just need to know. They phoned me to say that Emily did not have Down's syndrome. From that point on I just relaxed and enjoyed the rest of the pregnancy.

> *I felt confident – I could see where the needle was and where the baby was*

## No, I refused the amnio test

### Diana, 36, and baby Daisy

I think that we were quite lucky during the pregnancy. The midwife who looked at me was very good at talking about the different tests that were possible and what they might show. This meant that early on in the pregnancy, I had a sickle-cell anaemia test. This test was important for us as we are both black, and I needed to be checked to see if I was a carrier. We also both knew people who had had it. It is a really painful condition and I wouldn't have wanted a child to be born with it.

Later on in the pregnancy, I was offered an amniocentesis, but after talking it through with Rob, I decided not to have it. I don't like needles and you don't get the results back until quite late on. While I probably would have had a termination early on for sickle-cell anaemia, there is no way that I would have had a late termination. I also didn't want to worry about waiting for the results and so I just took my chances. Our midwife was great and didn't try and make us change our minds. I did have my scans, though and I was really pleased that I did. One scan picked up that Daisy had one kidney that was not working properly and that means that they are now keeping checks on her progress.

In some ways deciding which tests to have or not to have is hard. I think that it is quite a personal decision and you do need to think about what you are letting yourself in for. We were given good advice and help from our midwife and I think that that really helped us.

> *Our midwife was great and didn't try and make us change our minds*

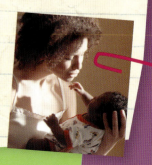

# Antenatal classes

Antenatal classes are a key part of your pregnancy care. While your antenatal appointments monitor you, your pregnancy and your baby, antenatal classes take a more general look at what happens in childbirth and beyond. They give you a chance to explore your feelings about your pregnancy and the future.

Your midwife or doctor will let you know about the free classes run by the NHS. These do fill up quickly, so book in early. Other classes are available, but you may need to pay for these.

## Early booking

Classes start about 10 weeks before your baby is due, so remember to put your name down well before that time to avoid disappointment.

## Meet a mate

Antenatal classes are a great way to meet other women, compare pregnancies and find answers to your questions and worries. And you find that you are not alone. Friendships you make in antenatal classes will often last well beyond the birth of your babies.

### Top tip

If you just want to listen in a class, that's fine. If you want to ask loads of questions, that's fine too.

**Did you know?** Antenatal classes are sometimes called parentcraft classes.

*You may think:*
- **I don't have time**
- **I've already read about everything I'll hear in class**
- **My friends have told me all I need to know**
- **I know exactly what I want for the birth**
- **It's all too scary. I don't want to know**

*Well, you're wrong!*
- **Antenatal classes usually only last for an hour or two. If they are in work time, your employer is legally required to give you time off to attend**
- **You may think you've read about all the options open to you, but nothing beats the most up-to-date information**
- **Advice from friends and family is brilliant. But they don't know it all, and it may be a welcome relief to have clear up-to-date information from a professional such as a midwife**
- **Even if you know what you want for the birth, antenatal classes offer lots more information about exercises and other health tips to get you in the best shape possible for the birth and caring for your new baby. Finding out more about labour and the choices you have can make it feel less daunting**

*Top ten reasons to go to an antenatal class*
1. **Meet other mums-to-be and their partners**
2. **Hear the answer to those embarrassing questions you thought nobody else would ask**
3. **Find out how to care for a new baby**
4. **Find out more about relaxing**
5. **Have a tour of the labour ward**
6. **Find out more about labour**
7. **Find out more about pain relief and other ways to relax in labour**
8. **Receive some emotional support**
9. **See what equipment may be used during labour**
10. **Know that you're not the only person who feels this way**

*Topics covered in antenatal classes*
- **health in pregnancy**
- **coping with labour and birth**
- **pain relief in labour**
- **exercises during and after pregnancy**
- **relaxation**
- **feelings about the birth**
- **feelings about being a new mum or dad**
- **caring for your baby**
- **breastfeeding**
- **relationship changes with your partner**

### Choosing a class

Some classes focus on one or two particular topics, so it's a good idea to ask the teacher what she covers, to make sure it's the class for you.

### Time off from work

Legally you may take time off work (paid in most cases) to go to your antenatal classes. Your employer may ask to see a letter in which your midwife or doctor recommends these classes as part of your pregnancy care and confirms your attendance.

## National Health Service (NHS) classes

### Who runs them?

NHS classes are run by a health professional such as a midwife. They are often held in a hospital or health centre. Your midwife will tell you what classes are available in your area.

### When are they held?

Some NHS classes are in the daytime and others in the evening. It depends on what is available in your area.

### How long are they?

Classes are usually about one or two hours, and run as a course over several weeks.

### Labour ward

Some NHS classes offer a guided tour of the labour ward. This can make it less scary when you go to the ward in labour. If this tour isn't offered, ask and someone can arrange to show you around.

### Who can go?

Most classes welcome partners or friends for the whole course, but a few may only offer a couple of sessions for partners or friends.

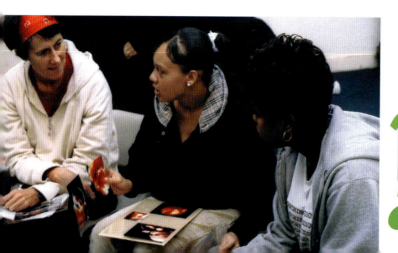

### Top tip

Find out about NCT antenatal classes early on (around weeks 10–12). They are popular, so you need to book early.

## Private antenatal classes

NHS classes are free, but classes are often quite big. Private classes are often smaller, so there is more time to go into detail and to ask lots of questions. You usually have to pay for private classes, although some teachers reduce their charges for people on low incomes. You can go to NHS and private classes, and get the best of both!

The National Childbirth Trust (NCT) (address, page 106) runs some of the most popular smaller classes. Trained NCT antenatal teachers are experienced mums who usually hold the classes in their own homes.

### Refresher classes

If you already have a child, you may have forgotten everything, and things may have changed. Don't worry – ask your midwife about refresher classes to remind you about your options and think about how you will manage with more than one child.

### Intensive courses

In some areas, you can go to intensive courses called Labour Days or Labour Weekends. Some women prefer to find out all there is to know in one blast. For others, it's too intense! Ask your midwife if you are interested.

### "I'll feel out of place"

Perhaps you are a teenager mum-to-be and can't face being with older mums. You may feel as if you'll have nothing in common with them. You will – you are all having babies. There are classes especially for teenage mums – ask your midwife or doctor what's available in your area.

**left** Friendships you make in antenatal classes will last well beyond pregnancy and birth as you meet up again to share experiences and show off your new baby.

**Did you know?** The women at your antenatal classes should all be due around the same time, so you may bump into them on the labour ward or at clinics after your baby is born!

### "I'll be on my own"

Many women don't have a partner or choose to go to a class on their own. Some women take a friend who plans to be with them at the birth. Find out before you go if partners or friends are welcome.

### "What's in it for my partner?"

Your partner may not be physically giving birth but it will reassure them to know what to expect and how best to support you. A new baby is a major change in a relationship, and antenatal courses often cover how you can both adapt to the new arrival.

### Antenatal exercise classes

Antenatal exercise classes focus on exercises to keep you fit in pregnancy, to relax you and to prepare you for labour. They include:

- aquanatal classes held in a swimming pool (and yes, you have to get wet!)
- yoga
- Pilates
- relaxation

## Top tip

Before you sign up for a course of classes, find out if there is a particular focus to the course – for example, some classes emphasise labour without pain relief. This may suit you perfectly or you may prefer a class that covers all aspects of labour.

### Complementary therapies

There are many other ways to relax and prepare your body and mind for labour. Some women find osteopathy or chiropractic (gentle manipulation), hypnosis and other complementary therapies helpful. Some treatments aren't safe in pregnancy so make sure your teacher or practitioner:

- belongs to an accredited professional association (see page 106)
- is qualified to treat women in pregnancy
- knows you are pregnant!

## We giggled a lot!

**Antenatal classes are a great way to meet new friends who are just as excited as you – and as scared – about being pregnant and giving birth. Diane (22) made lots of new friends when she was pregnant with Sam.**

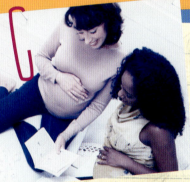

I really enjoyed going to antenatal classes when I was pregnant. I started going when I was about 28 weeks pregnant and we had six sessions in all, which were held at the hospital. I was a bit nervous about going to the classes as I didn't know anyone but I quickly found another woman to team up with. Everyone was friendly and we had plenty of time to chat and get to know each other.

I made a lot of friends and we still meet up which is great for me, as before the class I didn't know any other new mums. It's nice now to be able to pick up the phone or visit someone else's house who is going through the same thing and to have a moan or a laugh.

Every week was about something different – I found the session about giving birth particularly useful. We giggled a lot and talked through some of our fears. I liked the way that we could ask questions and sometimes other people's questions were ones that I had wondered about too. We also looked at feeding the baby and things we would need straightaway. I hadn't really thought about how I

was going to feed the baby up until that session and I hadn't bought any nappies or packed a bag ready to go into hospital. You tend when you are pregnant only to think as far as the birth.

On one of the last sessions, we went around the labour ward. That was really interesting and when it came to giving birth, I felt that I knew my way around and I even recognised a couple of members of staff. Later on the ward, I also saw a couple of women who had been in the class with me. It was lovely to catch up with them and meet their new babies. I'd been worried about getting the time off work, because even though I knew it was my right to go, I wasn't sure about it. My employer was great though and, looking back, the classes were certainly worth going to. I would have really missed out on a lot of information and new friends, if I had not gone.

*Every week was about something different*

# All change – half way there!

The second part of pregnancy often feels like the easiest. Many niggles from the early weeks have disappeared and you are not yet so big that it feels uncomfortable. It's a time when many women blossom and enjoy the pregnancy.

## Top tip

Being pregnant is no excuse not to wear a seat belt. Put the lap belt under your bump and the shoulder belt between your breasts.

## Check this out

Check out pages 12 and 61 for more information about complaints which are common in early and late pregnancy – many women experience these amazing variety of physical niggles and problems at different times and even throughout their pregnancy.

## Common physical problems

If you feel unwell or have any of the symptoms listed on page 35, don't delay. See a doctor or midwife as soon as possible, or get someone to take you to a hospital.

| Problem | Why? | Top tips |
|---|---|---|
| **Backache** | Your bump is growing and your muscles are relaxing – not a great combination for your back. | • Check out the posture ideas on page 91 to make sure that you stand tall and protect your back when lifting.<br>• Try to de-stress, even if it's just taking a few minutes to breathe slowly and deeply. If you feel all tense, your body will tense and then it's more likely to feel uncomfortable or to seize up.<br>• Avoid lifting heavy objects.<br>• Make sure you bend your knees when you lift. Make your thighs do the work, and squat down before you lift.<br>• Sit tall – make sure your chair is comfortable, especially if you work at a desk.<br>• Take some gentle exercise, such as swimming or yoga.<br>• Avoid lifting from a height as it's easy to lose your balance.<br>• Encourage toddlers to walk whenever possible.<br>• Avoid high heels!<br>• Carry weights evenly (so carry a shopping bag in each hand, rather than one very heavy bag in just one hand). |
| **Breasts leaking** | • Don't worry – your milk is not about to suddenly gush through while you are in a meeting.<br>• This is a form of milk called colostrum, and your body is busy in preparation to feed your baby. | If you need to, wear a breast pad. |

| Problem | Why? | Top tips | Seek medical help |
|---|---|---|---|
| **Swelling (oedema)** | If your rings feel a bit tight or your shoes a bit uncomfortable, this is probably due to the increased amount of fluids in your body. Swelling or puffiness is most noticeable in hands and feet. | • Avoid tight shoes or clothes.<br>• Drink plenty of water (it will help flush out the excess fluid).<br>• Avoid standing for long periods.<br>• Sit with your legs slightly raised.<br>• Mention it to your doctor or midwife at your next visit. | • If the swelling is extreme and you also have headaches or blurred vision, contact your doctor or midwife as soon as possible. This could be a sign of a potentially dangerous condition called pre eclampsia (see page 58).<br>• If you have a sore swelling on your leg, contact your doctor or midwife as soon as possible as this could be a sign of a blood clot, which needs to be treated immediately. |
| **Leaking bladder** | Your growing uterus is pushing down on your bladder so you may find that when you laugh or cough, you leak a bit of wee. | • Remember your pelvic floor exercises (see page 9).<br>• Don't cut back on fluid intake – this is dangerous for the baby.<br>• Wear a light pad, avoid lifting heavy objects and go for a wee when you need to.<br>• Mention it to your doctor or midwife at your next visit so she or he can check there is no infection.<br>• If the leaking is prolonged, wear a clean sanitary pad and check it 20 minutes later. | • If the pad is still damp, contact your midwife or as she will probably want to check that your waters haven't broken.<br>• If the pad is a pinkish brown or green colour, take it in with you.<br>• Meanwhile, write down the time and put on another pad. |
| **Constipation** | As hormones relax your muscles, including those responsible for bowel movement, they don't work as well as they did before you were pregnant. | • Eat plenty of fibre-rich foods, especially fruits and vegetables.<br>• Drink plenty of water – aim for 8 glasses a day.<br>• Take some gentle exercise – such as walking or swimming. | Speak to your doctor or midwife if prolonged or painful, or if you experience constipation while taking iron tablets. |
| **Heartburn** | Stomach acid leaks out of the top of the valve into your stomach. This feels like a burning in the chest. | • Eat little and often, and avoid spicy foods.<br>• A milky drink can help too. | If this doesn't work, speak to your midwife or doctor who will be able to prescribe you something. |
| **Heat** | Your body is working much harder to move around and nourish your baby. | • Keep cool.<br>• Drink plenty of water.<br>• Stay out of the sun. | If you feel faint or dizzy speak to your doctor or midwife. |
| **Haemorrhoids (piles)** | Swollen veins round your anus. They look like grapes and feel itchy and sore. Often worse if you are con-stipated. | • Follow the top tips (above) to avoid constipation.<br>• Apply a haemorrhoid cream, which you can get from your chemist. | See your doctor if piles are too uncomfortable or if there's any bleeding. |
| **Bleeding gums** | Hormonal changes make gum disease more likely. | • Try to avoid sugary foods.<br>• See your dentist if you haven't already.<br>• Brush gently. | |
| **Food craving** | Hungry for particular foods, or strange combinations? It's quite natural. | Don't use as an excuse to eat unhealthy food. | If you crave non-food items, talk to your midwife. |

| Problem | Why? | Top tips | Seek medical help |
|---|---|---|---|
| **Thrush** | This is a fungal infection of the vagina and can be more frequent in pregnancy. You may have a thick white vaginal discharge (it looks a bit like cottage cheese) and maddening itching around your vagina. | • You can get pessaries or cream from the chemist – tell the pharmacist you are pregnant.<br>• Mention it to your midwife or doctor at your next visit – if they prescribe the treatment you can get it free. | See your doctor if you have a vaginal discharge that is brown, red or green, and/or smells bad. |
| **Varicose veins** | These are bulging dark veins in your legs caused by the increased blood supply. | • Avoid standing for long periods.<br>• Wear support tights.<br>• Lie with your feet slightly raised.<br>• Circle your ankles one way and then the other to keep your circulation going.<br>• Don't cross your legs. | If you have a sore swelling on your leg, contact your doctor or midwife as soon as possible as this could be a sign of a blood clot, which needs to be treated immediately. |
| **Stress** | Maybe you are worried about your pregnancy, your relationship, your job, or money. | Take some time out from your anxieties to close your eyes and relax. Even 10 minutes a day can make a huge difference to you, and to your baby. Talk to your partner or a friend or relation. Sometimes just talking about it can help. | If this doesn't work, speak to your midwife or doctor who will be able to prescribe you something. |

**Check this out** See page 84 for advice on healthy eating.

*Did you know?* Many niggly problems you have can be helped at work! When your boss does a risk assessment, he or she should, as appropriate
• provide you with a supportive chair
• make sure you have easy access to a loo
• make sure you have easy access to drinking water or can take breaks to get a drink
• make sure you don't spend too long standing

**right** Try to make some time every day to relax. Turn off the TV, take the phone off the hook, put your feet and close your eyes. Fast forward to a time when you are holding your beautiful new baby. Sing to your baby if you like – he can hear you! Even 10 minutes of relaxation a day can make a huge difference – to you and your baby.

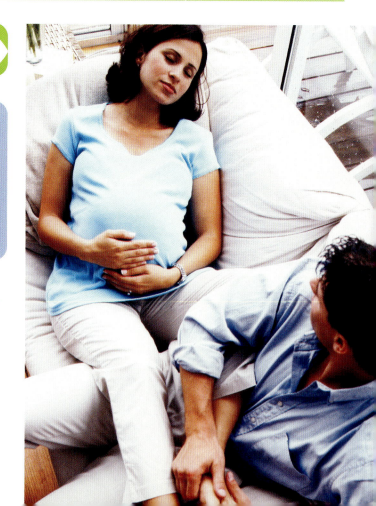

# Where will I have my baby?

Choosing where to give birth is a big decision. You'll be asked where you would like to give birth at your booking appointment. You may want time to think about it before deciding, and you can always change your mind at any time. If you'd like more information or more time to decide, ask your midwife or doctor.

## Places you might give birth:

**In hospital** – in a specialist unit where obstetricians are on duty as well as midwives. You may be advised to give birth in hospital if your pregnancy needs special care (see page 95).

**At home** – your midwife will stay with you during labour and birth.

**In a doctor's or midwife unit** – this may be part of a large hospital, a small community hospital or completely separate.

> *Your choices may be limited if:*
> - **you are having twins or more**
> - **you or your baby has a medical condition that needs to be monitored**
> - **you had problems in a previous pregnancy.**

Don't be afraid to ask questions – doctors and midwives usually have good practical reasons for these decisions. For example, your community team may not have enough midwives to offer home births, your hospital unit might be short-staffed or your consultant may want you closer to hospital if there is an emergency.

### *Why choose hospital birth?*
- ✓ **specialist teams and equipment on hand if you need it**
- ✓ **anaesthetist available if you want an epidural**
- ✓ **midwives on hand to help you and your baby get into a routine**
- ✓ **visiting hours help you to rest**
- ✓ **a break from other children, if you have them**

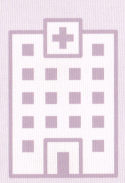

### *Why choose home birth?*
- ✓ **familiar, comfortable surroundings**
- ✓ **no need to be away from young children**
- ✓ **more privacy**
- ✓ **you don't have to fit into a hospital routine**
- ✓ **a strong relationship with the midwife who will be with you for the delivery**

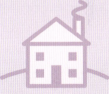

### *Why choose a small maternity unit?*
- ✓ **usually quite informal and relaxed**
- ✓ **rooms often decorated to look more like home than hospital**
- ✓ **easy access to essential equipment**
- ✓ **if it is on the same site as a hospital, it is easy to transfer you if there is a problem**

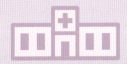

## Q&A

**Q.** Can I have a water birth?

**A.** Check with your doctor or midwife what is available in the hospital or community unit.

**Q.** What type of pain relief can I have for a home birth?

**A.** You can use TENS and Entonox (gas and air) (see page 65) but you can't have an epidural at home.

**Q.** Can my partner be there?

**A.** Yes, your partner or a friend can be with you wherever you give birth.

**Q.** Can I move around in labour?

**A.** Yes, this is encouraged unless there are medical reasons for you not to as it will help you manage the pain and find positions which are most comfortable for you.

**right** If everything is going well with your pregnancy, a water birth may be possible. Ask what is available in your hospital or community unit or – if you want a home birth – about hiring a pool. Just relaxing in a warm bath can help ease the pain of labour.

**Q.** Can I choose music to listen to?

**A.** You can usually take a choice of music – check in advance if there is any equipment for playing your favourite CDs or cassettes, or whether you need to take in your own equipment, which should be battery-operated.

**Q.** Do I have to breastfeed if I'm in hospital?

**A.** The nurses and midwives will encourage you to try because of the benefits to you and your baby. But if you cannot or feel strongly that you don't want to, they will help you bottle feed.

**Q.** How soon can I go home?

**A.** If you have a straightforward delivery, and you and your baby are both well, you can go home after a few hours. If you have a caesarean, you will need to stay in hospital for a few days.

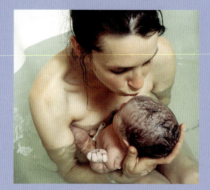

**Q.** How long can I stay for?

**A.** Many new mums choose to stay in for at least a night to recover their energy. Many second-time mums choose to stay in for at least a night to have some rest from the demands of other children!

**Q.** Can my baby stay in bed with me if I'm in hospital?

**A.** This is not recommended for any woman, at home or in hospital. You may be so exhausted from the labour that it can put your baby at risk from being squashed or suffocated. Sleeping in the same bed as your baby is not recommended at all for the first 6 months, and especially not if either you or your partner smoke. The best is to have your baby sleeping In his own cot in your room for the first six months.

**Q.** Will there be someone who can show me what to do?

**A.** There'll be plenty of qualified people in hospital to show everything from bathing your baby to changing her nappy! If you give birth at home, your midwife will stay for a couple of hours. After you have your baby (wherever that is) a community midwife continues to see you at home or in hospital to make sure you and your baby are OK. If you need help, do ask.

If you have a question that isn't answered here, call Tommy's pregnancy information line on **0870 777 30 60** and speak to one of our experienced midwives.

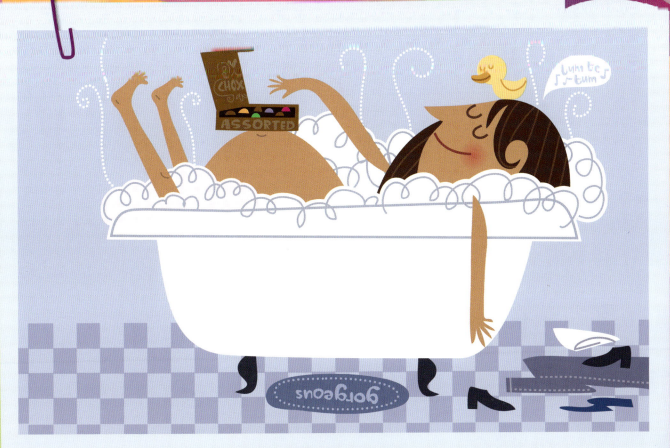

**Q.** I am terrified that I will get stretch marks. What can I do to prevent them?

**A.** Stretch marks are a bit of a lottery in pregnancy and often depend on your skin type. Your skin has to cover more surface area and stretch marks usually appear on the abdomen, thighs and breasts. At first they are red and are very noticeable; after pregnancy, they shrink down and fade away to a silvery colour. Some women use moisturisers and creams as a preventive measure, but there are no absolute guarantees that they work. Excessive weight gain can also cause stretch marks so a healthy diet can help (see page 84).

**Q.** Now I am pregnant, women I barely know come up to me and tell me how awful their experience was. This is making me really scared.

**A.** Don't let other women offload their baggage on you. Just tell them when your baby is due, that you are feeling fine – and then make it clear that you are not interested in birth stories.

If you have been scared by stories you've heard, learn about your options for pain relief in labour, and talk to your midwife about any worries you have.

**above** Your body works hard to be pregnant, so try and spend some time relaxing each day. A warm bath, candles, music and someone to talk to can all help you wind down.

**Q.** I know I shouldn't worry about the pregnancy, but I can't stop myself. Everyone tells me to stop worrying and enjoy it.

**A.** If you feel that your body is controlling you and not the other way around, take control! Gentle exercise, healthy diet and relaxation can help you take charge of your body.

### Top tip

You can start your baby's photo album now! Ask to have a copy of the picture of your baby from your first and following scans. You may need to pay a little for this.

If you have a question that isn't answered here, call Tommy's pregnancy information line on **0870 777 30 60** and speak to one of our experienced midwives.

53

# Not long to

These are the last few weeks of your pregnancy. It is an exciting time, as the end is in sight. You'll start packing bags and getting ready for birth, and getting the clothes and equipment you will need for your baby's first weeks. This section tells you what to expect and helps you prepare for the birth.

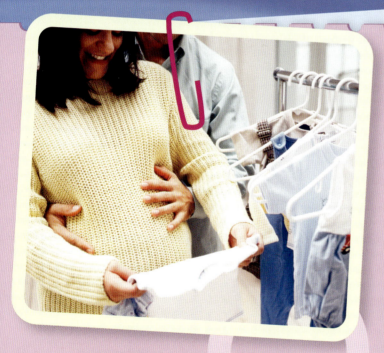

**above** You may enjoy shopping for lots of baby clothes and equipment, or you may prefer to wait for your baby to arrive. People will give you toys and clothes so it's a good idea to buy just the basics until you know what exactly you need.

## Weeks 29-40

Your baby continues to grow, and from now on has a better chance of survival if he is born early. You will visit your midwife more often for checks on you and your baby's health. The position your baby is lying in becomes more important and you may start to think about what happens in labour.

Women's feelings about this stage of pregnancy can vary enormously. You may feel that time is dragging on slowly, and long for a time when you don't feel so tired. Or you may find that these last few weeks give you time to get ready for the baby and to enjoy some time for yourself, especially after you start maternity leave.

Below is a guide for this part of the pregnancy. You might find that exact timings for antenatal care appointments are different in your area. This calendar is only a guide to what is happening to you and your baby. Don't worry if things don't exactly follow this pattern. Each woman and each baby is different.

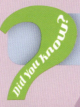
*Did you know?*

A baby born before 37 weeks is referred to as 'premature'.

# go now!

| | Your baby's development | Your body | Healthy tips | Things to do/ that happen | How you may feel |
|---|---|---|---|---|---|
| **weeks 29-30** | Your baby will measure approximately 42cm from top to toes. His fingers and fat layers are forming.<br><br>Her eyelids open and she can even respond to light outside the uterus. | You may suffer from varicose veins.<br><br>If you wear them, contact lenses may feel dry.<br><br>Your belly button may stick out a bit. This will go back to its usual shape after the birth.<br><br>You may feel breathless as you breathe harder for you and your baby. | Put your feet up when you can. Wearing support tights can help.<br><br>If your contact lenses make your eyes feel dry, talk to your optician, who might recommend eye drops.<br><br>Take lots of rest. | Pack your labour and baby bag (see page 69).<br><br>Check you have all the basic baby equipment you need – the rest can wait until you and your baby go on a shopping trip!<br><br>Week 29 of your pregnancy is the earliest you can start your maternity leave.<br><br>Give a colleague at work, or a friend, a list of emergency contacts, just in case. | You may be feeling anxious about the labour and birth and may start to have vivid dreams about the birth (see page 62).<br><br>Try to make some time for you and your partner if you have one. |

| | Your baby's development | Your body | Healthy tips | Things to do/ that happen | How you may feel |
|---|---|---|---|---|---|
| **weeks 31-32** | If your baby is born prematurely, he has a good chance of survival – he can take air into his lungs and breathe properly, although he would still need some specialist care. | You may feel your uterus tighten and harden for a few seconds. These painless movements are Braxton Hicks contractions (see page 62). If you experience a dramatic increase of vaginal discharge, or a significant leaking of what you think is wee, check with your midwife. She or he can check if your waters have broken. | Make sure you lift things correctly, to prevent backache. (see page 91). | Keep talking and singing to your baby. She can hear you and may recognise your voice after the birth! Antenatal classes start around now. Start thinking about your birth plan (see page 67). | You may feel clumsy, and off-balance, so take care if you are riding a bicycle, or stepping on or off a bus or train. |
| **weeks 33-36** | If this is your first baby she may move down into your pelvis, ready for birth. When it has pushed down a certain amount it is called 'engaged'. If your baby does not move into a head-down position, your obstetrician may recommend trying to push the baby around with his/her hands. | Your breasts will feel heavier. You may find it difficult to get comfortable to sleep. And when you do, you may need to get up to have a wee. If you are expecting twins or more you will probably have your babies very soon! Hormones relax the pelvic joints in preparation for birth so you may feel a few aches and pains in your pelvis. | Rest whenever you can. Keep drinking lots of water. Rock back and forth gently on the loo to make sure you empty your bladder. | If you are planning to breastfeed, it's a good idea to be measured for a feeding bra and buy a couple in advance. Don't plan air travel as many airlines won't take women in late pregnancy. If you have other children, make arrangements for someone to look after them when you go into labour. Think about how you will get to the hospital or unit where you plan to give birth. Practise some positions for labour with your birth partner (see page 75). | You may start to feel excited that your baby's about to arrive. This is a good time to double check that you're ready to go! Have you packed everything you need? (see page 69) |
| **weeks 37-40** | Your baby is putting on 28g (1oz) a day. There's not much room to kick now, so it's just wriggles from now on. Your baby may be ready for birth any time now! | When your baby engages, you may feel less breathless. This is called 'lightening'. Twins or not, you are considered full-term now, so be prepared … | Look out for signs of labour (see page 72). | If this is your first baby, you may have weekly antenatal appointments from week 37. Make sure the car is filled with petrol or you have the telephone numbers of reliable taxi firms. | You may start to feel restless. You may feel the urge to 'nest' but try to avoid the temptation to paint your kitchen a new colour. It's time to rest now. |

# An obstetrician's day

Dr Louise Kenny is an obstetrician in a unit that specialises in complicated pregnancies, including high blood pressure, pre-eclampsia and kidney problems.

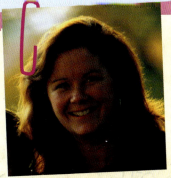

My working day starts with a visit to the antenatal ward. This is the ward where expectant mums stay if there are complications in their pregnancies. Our unit specialises in women who have high blood pressure, pre-eclampsia or kidney problems, and often the mums are a long way from home. I try my best on these visits rounds to be cheery as it is hard for women who can get fed up of waiting around and feel quite homesick.

Medical students are usually with me as we check up on each of the women. We try to make it as informal as possible and chat to women. For the medical students it is a really important way to learn. Books and lectures can't give them the first-hand experiences that will eventually make them into good doctors.

I then normally go down to antenatal clinic. We have a morning clinic for routine antenatal care and another more specialised clinic in the afternoon, where I see women with high blood pressure and kidney problems. Our clinic gets really busy. We see around 60–70 women in the morning and we have four or five doctors on. It is a balancing act to try to make sure every woman gets enough time. Having myself sat in waiting rooms for three hours at a time, I know how tedious it can be. Bringing a friend, partner or relative along can be a good idea, especially if units offer an early ultrasound on the booking visit.

Once the morning antenatal clinic is over, I try to grab something to eat before the afternoon session starts. I also catch up with paperwork, letters from doctors and look over any test results that might have come in.

We see fewer women in the afternoon, but we are still busy, as we need to spend more time with them. They might have had a complicated previous pregnancy or have a pre-existing medical condition. This is often quite challenging work as we are trying to maintain the woman's health and get the best outcome for the baby.

*Keeping an open mind about what you'll need in labour is a good idea.*

My own two pregnancies were each very different. My first was straightforward and uncomplicated. For my second I had an emergency caesarean section and a pre-term baby. I think that, like all women, I started with certain ideas about how labour and birth would go, but you have to be ready to roll with what happens sometimes. Keeping an open mind about what you'll need in labour is a good idea. Sometimes it will all go better than expected and other times it might not go to plan.

*I try my best to be cheery as women can get fed up of waiting around – and quite homesick.*

The afternoon clinic finishes around five and I try to get back on to the antenatal ward again before catching up with paperwork and then going home. On some days, I am on call and will stay in the hospital and be up on the labour ward through the night. On a typical night on call, I would expect to deliver a couple of births by forceps, ventouse or caesarean. Where labours are going well, the midwifery team handle everything, and they only call us in when they have some concerns. I only go in if the labour has stopped or if the baby is showing signs of distress.

I usually phone home at around half past eight to check that the kids have eaten, done their homework and, of course, to tell them I love them. They have always had a working doctor mum although if it were not for my own mum, it would be hard to juggle everything. I love my job. I've been delivering babies for over 10 years and I sometimes still have a little cry when a new baby arrives. It is such a special moment in women's lives and being part of that moment is a real privilege.

# Antenatal care - Final weeks

**E**xtra checks in these last three months help your midwife to reassure you that all is well - or deal early with any problems so that you can look forward to a safe and happy delivery.

From week 28 you will have more frequent antenatal appointments. From week 36 your midwife will also check on your baby's position.

**28 weeks** Check the size of your abdomen, test urine, measure blood pressure.

**32 weeks** Check the size of your abdomen, test urine, measure blood pressure.

**34 weeks** Check the size of your abdomen, test urine, measure blood pressure. Second anti-D treatment if you are rhesus negative.

**36 weeks** Check the size of your abdomen, test urine, measure blood pressure.

**40 weeks** Check the size of your abdomen, test urine, measure blood pressure.

**41 weeks** Check the size of your abdomen, take a urine test and measure your blood pressure. Discuss your options for starting off labour.

## Keep your appointments

It's important not to miss any antenatal appointments in these final weeks. If you do have a problem, your antenatal team can spot the warning signs early and take action straight away.

*Your doctor and midwife are particularly on the lookout now for signs of:*
- **pre-eclampsia**
- **low-lying placenta**
- **breech or another 'wrong' position**

## Pre-eclampsia

Pre-eclampsia is a condition that can be dangerous for mum and baby. One of the signs of pre-eclampsia is an increase in blood pressure. Another is a high level of protein in the urine. Your midwife can measure both of these. This is why you need to keep your antenatal appointments.

*Other signs of pre-eclampsia include:*
- **bad headaches**
- **blurred vision or lights flashing before the eyes**
- **bad pain between the ribs**
- **sudden swelling of the face, hands or feet**
- **vomiting**

### *Top tip*

Now that you are in the final weeks, you may have many questions about the birth. Feel free to ask your midwife – she or he is the expert and is there to help you.

## Low lying placenta

Low-lying placenta (also called placenta praevia) is a condition where the placenta lies below the baby in the uterus, covering the cervix. If your 18–23 week scan showed your placenta was low, you will be offered another scan at 30 weeks. This will show if the placenta has moved upwards. If it stays low, and is still covering the cervix, the baby cannot safely be delivered vaginally, so you may need a caesarean.

## Wrong way up!

Not all babies get into a head-first position for delivery. They may position themselves

- bottom-first ('breech')
- sideways
- diagonally
- or even feet first

If your baby is not facing head down your midwife or doctor may try gently to push your baby around your tummy into a head-first position. This is called 'external cephalic version' (ECV). But some babies are just too comfy where they are, and won't budge – so it doesn't always work!

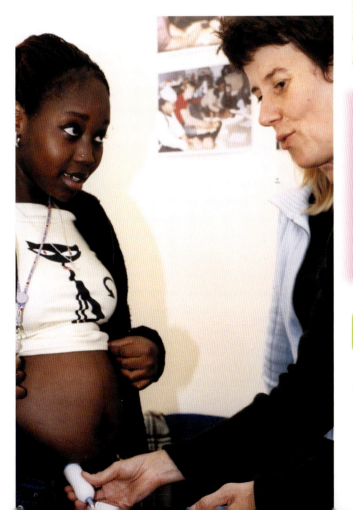

**Top tip**

Take time to get to your antenatal classes. They really are worth it

*Questions you may want to ask*
- **"Is my baby in the right position?"**
- **"Is she the right size for the dates?"**
- **"How will I know when I'm in labour?"**
- **"I'm getting worried about being a mum"**
- **"Are these Braxton Hicks contractions (see page 62) or the real thing?"**

**Top tip**

If you are feeling unsure about where you have chosen to have your baby, you can always change your mind. Talk it through with your doctor or midwife.

*Last few weeks!*
- **Your body has a way of signalling that your labour is coming soon**
- **Braxton Hicks contractions may get stronger (see page 62)**
- **You may lose weight a couple of weeks before the birth**
- **You may have a strong urge to bake bread or be homely, sorting out cupboards that you haven't bothered with for years – this is called 'nesting'**
- **You may have a sudden burst of energy.**

**Check this out**  Check out page 72 for signs of labour.

**left**  Your midwife listens to your baby's heartbeat at every appointment from around week 16.

# Get to know your baby

This is a great time to 'talk' to your baby. He's alert, can hear your voice, and can even detect light from outside the womb. Julie, 26, tells how she was in touch with her baby Jake even before he was born.

"

As my 'bump' grew I couldn't help touching and stroking it – it just seemed a natural way to protect the space around me and my baby.

I read an article that said that the unborn baby can hear from about 24 weeks onwards. I liked the idea that I could start to talk to my baby. I tried to make some quiet times when I could relax. Lying in the bath was best, I stroked my tummy and found myself singing 'Evergreen'. Well I've got a lousy voice and I don't even like Will Young, but my baby didn't seem to mind!

I played my Robbie Williams CDs over and over to my baby while I was relaxing. He joined in with a little kick now and then. I liked to imagine him dancing in there. Jake is now 11 months, nearly walking, and he loves holding my hands and bouncing to my favourite music.

My partner Sean joined in, talking and singing to my bump. He felt a bit silly at first, but I said it was just between us and he didn't have to tell his mates! One evening, Sean and I were having supper with some friends, and Jake gave me a huge kick – I think he wanted to join in our conversation!

Towards the end of my pregnancy, Jake was dancing all over the place, especially when I was trying to get to sleep. I tried to focus on the movements and gently stroke him and talk to him. Eventually he would stop dancing and I could get some sleep.

*I liked to imagine my baby dancing in there*

"

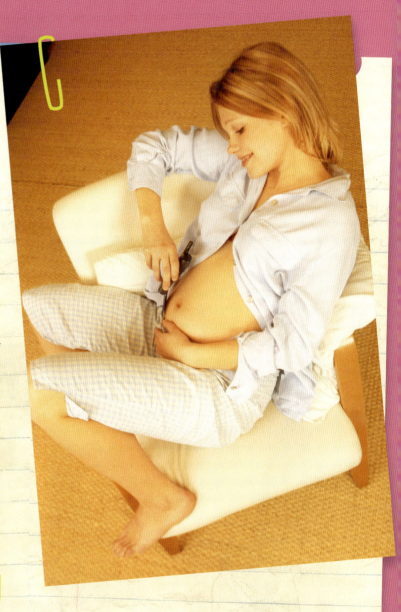

**above** Talking to your unborn baby can help you both to bond, you might even find that your baby responds to your voice after a while.

# All change – how your body prepares for birth

**N**early there! This last part of pregnancy is exciting, tiring and can feel scary too. You may feel very large now and your bump may make it hard to do up a shoelace, let alone get a good night's sleep. Your feelings may be all over the place – anxious but excited. Talk to other mums-to-be at your antenatal classes – you'll be surprised how many others feel just like you!

## Common physical problems

If you feel unwell or have any of the symptoms listed on page 35, don't delay. See a doctor or midwife as soon as possible, or get someone to take you to a hospital.

| Problem | Why? | Top tips | Seek medical help |
|---|---|---|---|
| **Abdominal pain** | Your growing uterus is stretching your tummy muscles. | Talk to your midwife about the difference between stretching pains and contractions. A warm bath may make you feel more comfortable. | If the pains are severe or there is any bleeding, seek medical help. |
| **Bleeding or spotting** | If it is jelly-like with red streaks it is a 'show' (see page 72). | If it's a show, it's probably nothing to worry about, but tell your doctor or midwife. | If there is bright red blood or constant spotting, contact your doctor immediately or ask someone to take you to the hospital. |
| **Rib pain** | This is due to your baby's position and kicking legs! | This pain will ease when your baby settles more into your pelvis area. | If you have severe pain between the ribs, like very bad heartburn – this may be a sign of pre-eclampsia (see page 58). |
| **Pelvis pain** | Your baby is getting into a position ready for birth. | The good news is once her head 'engages' or drops you may feel less breathless as there is more room for your diaphragm. | If the pain is severe, speak to your doctor or midwife. |
| **Finger pains!** | Even your fingers can suffer pregnancy niggles! If your fingers become numb or painful you may have carpal tunnel syndrome. This can affect women who need to make repetitive hand movements, like using a keyboard. | Give your hands a shake whenever you can and if you use a keyboard, try to keep your elbows above your wrists. | See your doctor if this is affecting your sleep or daily routine, they may suggest you see a physiotherapist. |
| **Itchiness** | Your skin may feel a bit itchy. It's the increased blood supply in your body. | If your skin is feeling a bit dry or itchy, you might try using a plain moisturiser without perfume. | If itchiness is severe, contact your doctor or midwife immediately as it may be a sign of a serious liver problem. |

| Problem | Why? | Top tips | Seek medical help |
|---|---|---|---|
| **Bad dreams** | Many women have dreams about their pregnancy, labour and baby. And these dreams can be nightmare-like. It doesn't mean everything is going to go wrong – it's a way of dealing with your fears and worries about the future that you may not express in your waking hours. | If you find yourself thinking and worrying about these dreams in the day, try to close your eyes and imagine positive images of you and your baby, with you holding and loving your baby. | |
| **Sleeplessness** | Your body is in overdrive, your baby has muddled up night and day and you keep needing to wee. No wonder it's hard to sleep. | Try not to fret about it, as that will make it more difficult. Have a milky drink before bed, and let your body just rest, even if you cannot sleep. Avoid caffeine, which is found in chocolate, coffee and fizzy drinks. | Ask your midwife for advice if it continues. |
| **Feeling uncomfortable** | You have a large bump, you are very tired and want to rest. But you can't get comfortable. | Take all the pillows you need to put them between your legs, under your head, wherever if feels better. Avoid lying on your back as the pressure from your baby can make you feel dizzy and can make piles even worse. | Ask your midwife for advice if it continues. |
| **Vaginal discharge** | You may notice an increase in your vaginal discharge due to structural and hormonal changes. | Wear cotton pants. Don't use a vaginal deodorant or a tampon. | If it is yellow, green, brown, itchy or smelly, contact your doctor or midwife as you may have an infection that is easy to treat. |

## Fact File

### Braxton Hicks contractions
From week 30 of your pregnancy, you may feel your tummy tighten for a few seconds. These are called Braxton Hicks contractions, and are not the start of labour. It's your body's way of preparing for the birth! See page 72 for signs of labour. Braxton Hicks contractions can be quite powerful and you can easily mistake them for labour contractions. If you are worried, phone your midwife or hospital for advice.

**Say again?** A 'show' is a small plug of jelly that blocks the entrance to your cervix while you are pregnant, It comes away as your cervix starts to stretch and get ready for the birth, usually after week 36. It may look blood stained but it is usually nothing to worry about.

## Top tip
Even if you feel ungainly, keep up with your exercise. Swimming is a great exercise at this stage. Even a brisk walk in the fresh air can refresh you and get your circulation going.

**Check this out** Check out pages 12 and 46 for more complaints common in early and mid pregnancy – many women experience physical problems at different times in their pregnancy.

# Thinking ahead –
## *pain relief*

Many women wonder how they will cope with the pain of childbirth. Everyone will deal with the experience in their own way. Some women find an inner calm that helps them focus – some want to swear and shout at their partners and some want all the pain relief they can have. Remember, it's not a competition! There are no prizes for the best performance during labour. Our guide gives you an outline of what pain relief is available. Your midwife can give you more information.

Until you're in labour, you might not know what you want. It's worth looking into your options – women who feel in control tend to have easier births. If you're stressed and tense, your contractions may feel more painful and become less effective, making your labour go on for longer.

### Be ready to have a change of plan
Not all women are the same. Not all births are the same, either. You may hear and read about other women's preferences for pain relief, but what is right or wrong for them may well be different for you.

During your labour, your needs might change. This is why many women try different positions and types of pain relief during their labour (see page 64). Do what feels best for you and don't feel bad if you change your mind.

### Learning about your body and how to relax
For centuries women in different parts of the world have used techniques such as acupuncture, hypnotherapy and aromatherapy to help with the pain of labour. If you are keen on giving birth without any medical pain relief, it is worth finding out what is available in your area well before your expected date.

Even if you think that you want medical pain relief during labour, it is worth learning about your body. Being able to relax rather than tense up during a contraction helps your body manage better. Many antenatal classes cover relaxation and breathing techniques – if this interests you, you might like to go to classes that concentrate on these techniques. Your midwife will know what is available in your area.

**right**  A female companion or doula may help you relax during labour.

**Say again?**  A doula is a woman who is trained to offer emotional and practical support to a woman (or couple) before, during and after childbirth.

### Being with the right person
Having the right person with you when you give birth can reduce the stress and therefore the pain. Think who will be good at making you feel relaxed and whom you most feel at ease with. Ideally, you want someone whom you can trust and who will be able to support you. This can be your partner, a relative or a friend. Some women hire a 'doula' who helps before, during and after the birth as a female support. Whoever you decide to be with, make sure that they understand that your needs and views may change during labour.

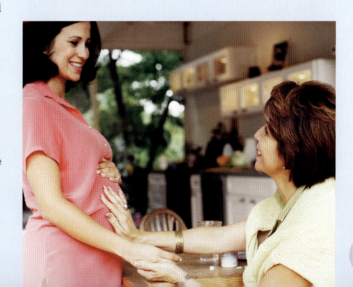

## Keep on moving

If you can, try and keep moving during the first stage of labour. This means that you are less likely to be tense. For the same reasons, you might want a massage or a back rub. Movement and massage help your brain to release its own pain-relieving chemicals called endorphins.

## Pain relief without drugs

| Method | How it works | How effective? | Advantages | Disadvantages | If you want this, tell your midwife in advance and … |
|---|---|---|---|---|---|
| **Breathing and relaxation exercises** | Slow, rhythmic breathing will set up a more relaxed state, which may help you cope better. | Effective for some women. | • Does not affect the baby. <br>• You are in control. <br>• Can be used alongside other pain relief. | • May require other pain relief or techniques alongside. | Find out about classes that will teach you techniques before the birth. |
| **Self-hypnosis** | Helps the body to reach a deep state of relaxation. | Effective for some women. | • Does not affect the baby. <br>• You are in control. <br>• Can be used alongside other pain relief. | • You need to learn and practise the techniques before the birth. <br>• May require other pain relief or techniques alongside. | Visit a qualified practitioner in plenty of time before the birth. |
| **Complementary therapies, eg Aromatherapy Reflexology Homeopathy** | Each of these works by using different stimulating agents, with the aim of achieving a relaxed state to help you cope better with labour. | Effective for some women. | • You are in control. <br>• Can be used alongside other pain relief. | • Some remedies not advisable, so you need to talk to a qualified practitioner who knows which remedies are safe. <br>• You will probably not be allowed to burn candles or essential oils in a hospital labour ward. <br>• May require other pain relief or techniques alongside. | Visit a qualified practitioner in plenty of time before the birth. They will need to accompany you at the birth with a certificate of qualification. |
| **Water** | A warm bath can help you relax in early labour even if you do not plan a water birth. | Effective for some women. | Does not affect the baby. Can be used alongside other pain relief. | • May not be available if the unit is busy. | Discuss whether you'd like a waterbirth with your midwife early in your pregnancy as special arrangements may need to be made. |
| **TENS (Transcutaneous Electrical Nerve Stimulation)** | A small machine, its pads attached to your lower back, sends out tiny electrical pulses which can get your body to produce pain-relieving endorphins. | Does not prevent pain completely. Some women find it more effective than others. | • You are in control of the levels. <br>• No effects on the baby. <br>• Can be used with other pain relief. | • You must begin to use it in early labour for maximum effectiveness. <br>• Not all women find it effective. <br>• Not used in bath or shower in case of electrocution. | • It is worth hiring or buying a machine so that you have it at the start of labour. <br>• Try out a machine first so that you can learn how it works. <br>• Use at the start of your labour. |

| Method | How it works | How effective? | Advantages | Disadvantages | If you want this, tell your midwife in advance and ... |
|---|---|---|---|---|---|
| **Entonox (gas and air)** | Using a mask, or mouthpiece you breathe in a mixture of nitrous oxide and oxygen at the start of – and during – a contraction. | Does not completely remove the pain, but takes the edge off it. | • You can use it at any time during labour. <br>• You are in control as to how often and when to use it. <br>• Easy to use. <br>• Does not affect your baby. | • Is a mild painkiller and does not remove all pain. <br>• May make your mouth feel dry. <br>• May make you feel sick. | • Use at the start of each contraction. <br>• Sip water or use ice cubes to keep your mouth moist. |
| **Pethidine** | A painkiller, related to morphine, that is given by injection. It makes you sleepy and relaxes the muscles of your uterus. | Takes some of the pain away, but not all. | • May help you to relax. | • Makes babies sluggish and drowsy, which can affect their breathing, feeding and your bonding. Takes around 4–5 days to clear from their systems. <br>• As it can make women feel and be sick, it is often combined with an anti-nausea drug. <br>• Cannot be used if you are towards the end of labour. <br>• May make you feel weepy and depressed. <br>• May slow labour down. <br>• Can make you feel drowsy and not in control. <br>• Later, your memory of labour may be a bit blurry. | • Find out in advance whether this is available in your hospital as not all units offer it. |
| **Epidural** | An anaesthetic inserted into the back, around the spine, through a needle. It blocks pain messages to the brain by deadening the nerves in the lower back. Dosage can be topped up as and when required throughout labour. | Very effective pain relief. | • Can offer complete pain relief for 90% of women. <br>• You can remain clear-headed. <br>• Brings down high blood pressure. <br>• If you are at a high risk of having a caesarean, you may not need extra anaesthetic. <br>• Does not affect the baby. | • You have less control over the delivery of your baby. <br>• It is more likely that you will need help to deliver the baby, such as forceps, ventouse or caesarean delivery (see pages 76 and 80). <br>• Epidurals cannot be offered for home births because they need to be given by an anaesthetist. <br>• Drips, monitor, catheters and numbness in your legs may mean that you may need to stay on the bed. <br>• May prolong labour. <br>• A very small number of women have a severe headache during and following the birth. | • Find out in advance if your hospital has anaesthetists on call to offer a 24-hour epidural service. <br>• Find out if you can have a mobile epidural that will allow you to move off the bed. <br>• If you are 8 or 9 centimetres dilated, and it's considered too late for an epidural, you will be offered alternatives. <br>• Lie still when the needle is inserted. <br>• Ask whether it can be left to wear off for the second stage of labour so that you can feel to push. |

### Wendy with Harry aged 3 months

## " I used pethidine and gas and air

Before the birth, you don't really know what to expect. But I did know that I didn't want an epidural. I didn't like the idea of having a needle put into my back or of losing feeling in my legs. I had the pethidine injection a few hours into the labour once the pain was building up. It didn't stop the pain, but looking back it probably took the edge off it.

Later, I had gas and air as well. I liked being able to hold the mask and was able to get the hang of taking in the gas and air before the contraction reached its peak. Even with the gas and air, I could still feel the pain, but I knew I could cope. I felt an inner strength that helped me to focus and concentrate. I know some women like to have their brows mopped, I just wanted to be left alone and deal with it in my own way. That's not to say that I wasn't pleased to have Mike there, but I just wanted a presence rather than someone talking to me. I think pain relief is quite a personal decision and no one can tell you what will or won't work. I know that other women hate pethidine, but for me it was fine. "

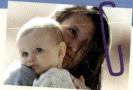

### Sarah with Ellen aged 8 months

## " I had an epidural

When I went into labour, I was already in hospital with high blood pressure. I think that constant monitoring brought it home to me that the way you give birth is far less important than having a healthy baby.

I didn't want pethidine – I didn't like the idea of an injection and unpredictable side effects. The labour was going well, but I needed some pain relief so I decided to have an epidural. They gave me a low dose and topped it up later. I still could feel the contractions and by the time it came for me to push it had nearly worn off so I could push my baby out.

I think that because I was realistic and knew that there was no way I could have a 'natural' birth I was more relaxed. We had calm relaxing music and dimmed the lights. It was not quite the birth I wanted, but it was still special. "

### Diane with Oliver aged 6 months

## " I didn't use any drugs

Before the birth, I looked at what was available and didn't fancy the idea of using drugs. The epidural was out for me because it involved needles, and pethidine was out because of its effects on the baby. Gas and air seemed a possible option, but I wasn't sure. I don't think that you can ever say 'never' before you know what it is like, so while I was hoping for a drug-free birth, I would have had something if I needed it.

I went to relaxation classes and bought a TENS machine. A friend had told me to try out the TENS machine at home beforehand and that was a good idea. I practised with it when I had some Braxton Hicks and got used to wearing it. When the contractions first started, I wasn't sure if they were for real as they were short and quite spaced out. As it was in the day, I decided to go for a walk nearby, although I did take my mobile with me just in case. I think that walking was good and it did take my mind off it. I also had a shower and pointed the spray head straight on to my back. That helped a lot.

Once the contractions became more serious, I phoned the hospital and went in. The TENS machine didn't stop the pain, but fiddling with the knob and having something to do and focus on was helpful. I also found that I could co-ordinate my breathing with it. It's hard to say if it stops the pain – because you have to concentrate so hard, you may not notice it so much. The other thing about being in labour is that time does go very quickly. When you hear about labour lasting for hours, you imagine agony for every second of every minute. But it is not like that. It felt more like tackling the surf of a wave and that is an image that I had in my head. I think having something to do during labour and being with the right person is probably just as important as the pain relief. "

# Thinking ahead – your birth plan

**G**iving birth is a hugely personal experience. Writing a birth plan is one way in which you can prepare for it. Making choices ahead of time is a good idea, because during labour itself, you might find it hard to concentrate or make a decision. It means that you'll think about issues like pain relief in advance – and not in the delivery room where you don't really have much time to think!

## What is a birth plan?

A birth plan is a list of your preferences during labour and birth. It can cover anything from your choice of pain relief to what happens immediately after your baby is born.

## Can I change my mind later?

A birth plan is not fixed. You might find on the day that you don't fancy a water birth or that you do want gas and air after all. Pain relief is one area where it is common to change your mind. Some women want to try to give birth without any medication, but during the birth change their minds. Others believe that they'll want an epidural early on, then find that they don't need anything!

## If I ask for something on a birth plan, can I be sure to get it?

A birth plan is about preferences not guarantees. No one can be 100% sure how your labour will go. Your midwife will try hard to respect your requests, but your health and that of your baby will always come first. Try to discuss your birth plan with your midwife during an antenatal visit as this can help you both.

Something you hope for might not be available. If another woman is in labour in the water pool, your hopes of a water birth might not be realised.

**below** A birth plan helps you to organise your ideas about the choices you have.

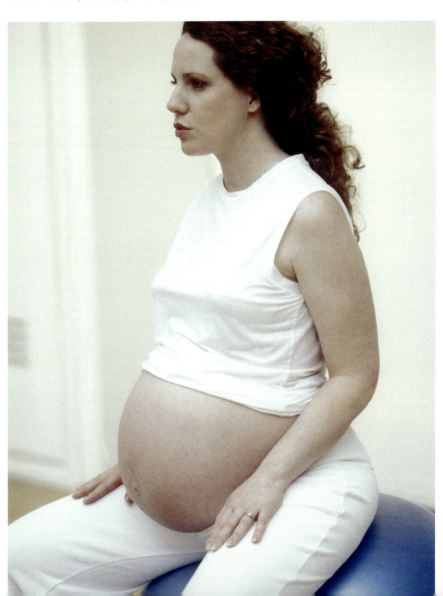

## Where can I get a birth plan?

Some health authorities have a birth plan template which you simply fill in. In other areas, you might have to draw up your own. Don't worry about it looking 'right'. There is no right way to write your birth plan. The main thing is to write down anything that you would definitely like to happen – or not happen. Your midwife will be happy to read it through with you and make any suggestions.

## I'm not very good at writing. Does it matter?

No. Once you have thought about your preferences, it is a good idea to talk them through with your midwife. You can always ask her to write them down if you are not sure about writing.

## What to include

**Birth partner:** Think who you'd like to be with you when you're in labour and what you'd like them to do.

**Atmosphere:** Think about the atmosphere you'd like to create. You could ask to take in music, have the lights dimmed or to use aromatherapy. And think about whether you'd mind if there were students present.

**Position and equipment:** Think about positions you would like to try (see page 75) and equipment you might need, such as a birthing stool, swiss ball, bean bag, water pool or TENS machine.

**Pain relief:** Think about what pain relief you might like (see page 64) if everything is going to plan. Then think what pain relief you might like if your labour is longer or more painful than you expect.

**above right** Your birth plan doesn't have to be very long – try to focus on the things that are really important to you.

### Top tip

- Give your midwife one copy of your birth plan.
- Keep another and have it with you when you go into labour.
- Talk your birth plan through with whoever is going to be with you on the day – make sure that they know that you might change your mind.
- Prepare to be flexible if things change during your labour.

### Birth plan for Jennifer Clark

- my date of birth 3 April 1981
- my baby's estimated due date 7 July 2005
- I would like Brian to support me, rub my back and cut our baby's umbilical cord
- I don't mind if one student midwife is there (not a group)
- I would like to try gas and air for pain relief. I would prefer not to have an epidural, but I will see how I feel at the time.
- I do not want my waters broken artificially unless it's necessary.
- I would like my baby placed straight on to my tummy after birth, and to have some quiet time with Brian and our baby as soon as possible.
- I don't mind having an injection to help deliver the placenta.
- Please call me Jenny
- I would like my partner Brian to be with me at the birth.
- I will bring in some favourite music for us both to listen to.
- I would like to try an active labour walking around in the early stages as much as possible, and to deliver my baby on all fours or upright.
- I do not want continuous monitoring of my baby's heart-beat unless it's necessary.
- I do not want an episiotomy unless in an emergency.
- I plan to breastfeed our baby and I would like some help getting started
- If all goes well I would like to go home after six hours.

**Medical intervention:** Your doctor or midwife may offer an intervention – something you cannot do yourself – to help your baby be delivered. You can find out more about these procedures on page 76. Before the birth, talk through them with your midwife, so that you can make a choice that you are happy with. But remember that on the day your choices might be limited because of the way the labour and birth are going.

# Thinking ahead – the kit you'll need

A few months ago, nine months was a long way off. But now with antenatal visits increasing and just a few days left to go, it is time to get ready for birth. We look at what you need to pack for yourself and your baby.

## Packing for labour and birth

You will need to pack a bag if you're going into hospital. You might give birth on your due date, but it's not a good idea to bet on this. Packing your bag now will mean that you have everything you want for your labour. As well as a bag ready for the birth, you'll need to pack some items for your stay and for your baby of course!

- Your antenatal notes: Make sure that you have your notes with you when you go to the hospital.
- An old, comfortable nightdress or t-shirt: make sure that it is cool and loose.
- Drinks and snacks: labour is a long haul, and if your partner stays with you they'll need food and drink too. Some partners faint because they haven't had enough food and water.
- Magazine or a book: some women find that they can keep themselves distracted in the early stages of labour with something to do or read.
- CDs or tapes and a player: make sure you have enough batteries.
- Face cloth and water: to keep you cool and fresh during labour.
- Camera: Check that you have enough film and a new battery.
- Change: for phone box and vending machines – you won't be able to use your mobile inside the hospital.
- Phone numbers: of family members and friends.

## Packing for your hospital stay

### For you
- Front opening nightdress.
- Light dressing gown and slippers.
- Hairbrush or comb.
- Toothbrush and paste.
- Favourite toiletries.

> " I made myself pack the bag one afternoon, but put it out of sight in a cupboard so I could forget about it. Packing the bag felt like a real step because it forced me to think about giving birth. "

- 24 Sanitary towels: for a few days following the birth, you will carry on bleeding as the uterus shrinks back to its original size. You will need extra absorbent sanitary towels. You cannot use tampons.
- Several pairs of pants.
- Two or three nursing or ordinary bras: your breasts will be much larger than usual.
- Breast pads: these absorb the leakage of first milk in the early days and you'll need them even if you do not intend to breastfeed.
- Clothes to come home in.

### For your baby
- Nappies.
- Vests and babygrows for the baby if you don't want to use hospital ones.
- Shawl or blanket.
- Baby socks.
- Baby hat.

## Ready at home

As well as packing bags for the hospital, you need to have a few things ready and waiting at home for the baby. Some women enjoy stocking up with lots of clothes and equipment, while others prefer to wait for the baby to arrive. Whatever your feelings, it's a good idea to have a basic 'start-up kit' ready, even if it stored at a friend's or relative's house. If money is tight, remember, not all items have to be brand new – except car seats and cot mattresses. Look out for things that you can borrow, or buy second hand, as long as they're clean and safe. People will give you toys and clothes as presents after the birth, so it's a good idea to buy just the basics until you know what exactly you need.

**below** Try to pack everything you need a few weeks before you're due to go into labour.

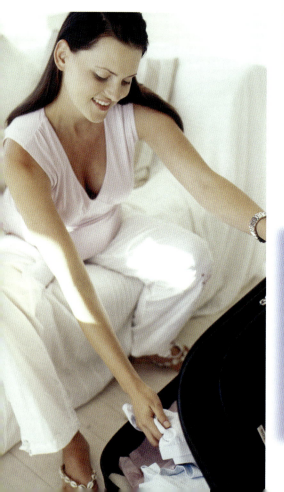

## Baby equipment

### Nappy changing
- Pack of nappies (new born size)
- Cotton wool
- Changing mat
- Barrier cream

### Bathing
- Washing up bowl or baby bath
- Clean soft towels

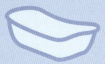

### Clothing
- Four all-in-one stretch babysuits
- Two cardigans
- Four vests
- Woolly hat, mittens and socks for cold weather
- Sunhat

### Sleeping
- Crib, carry cot or Moses basket
- Sheets
- Light blankets

### Breastfeeding
- Nursing bras (try on when you are around 36–38 weeks pregnant)
- Breast pads

### Bottle feeding
- Six bottles with teats and caps
- Sterilising equipment
- Bottle brush
- Infant formula milk

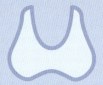

### Going out
- One or more of the following depending on how much space you have and whether you intend to make car journeys. If you are buying a new pram or pushchair, check whether you can fold it easily and how heavy it is.
- Baby carrier (sling)
- Car seat for a newborn
- Pram
- Pushchair with carrycot or reclining seat

## The nesting instinct

A couple of weeks before giving birth, some women find that they have an incredible urge to tidy and clean up their homes. They complete unfinished jobs around the home or suddenly feel desperate to clear out all the cupboards. If you feel this 'nesting' urge, take it easy! You need rest and safety – so if your project needs someone to go up a ladder, ask someone else to do it. Think about stocking up cupboards so that if you do not feel like going out you still have toilet rolls, washing powder and dried food.

> "Looking back, I bought far too much and many of the clothes were never even used as she was quite a big baby. I wish now that I had tried out different pushchairs once I had had her, as the one I got was quite heavy, even though it did look nice."

# Last-minute questions

## Q&A

**Q.** I'm starting to wonder whether I will be any good at being a mother. I've never been interested in children.

**A.** There are no medals when it comes to being a parent. Most of us just muddle our way through, getting some things right and a few things wrong along the way. Babies and children do not need perfect mothers. Your baby just needs you to take care of him, love and cuddle him. Talk through your fears with your midwife, your partner or a close friend.

**Q.** We have booked a holiday. I will be 30 weeks pregnant. Will I be able to fly?

**A.** Most airlines will let you fly providing you have a doctor's letter saying you are fit enough but check first. Book an appointment with your doctor to discuss your travel plans and don't forget to consider how many weeks pregnant you'll be at the end of your holiday if you need to fly back! If you are flying out of the country, check you have adequate travel and medical insurance. Remember to carry your notes with you. During the flight, avoid alcohol and drink plenty of water to prevent dehydration. It's a good idea to wear support stockings or socks on longer flights.

**right** Tell your partner how you're feeling.

**Q.** I am waking several times in the night. I am exhausted.

**A.** Some babies do bounce around at night and can press down on your bladder. This is tiring, but there is not too much that you can do about it. Try to go to bed a little earlier and experiment with sleep positions. As babies' sleep and waking routines alter during the pregnancy, you might even find that this is just a phase. If you cannot get back to sleep, try gently massaging your tummy and practise breathing and relaxing.

**Q.** My partner is excited about the baby, but he is getting over-protective.

**A.** It is great that your partner is keen to have a baby, but it must be irritating for you to be treated as if you were helpless. Tell your partner how you are feeling, and try to include him. There are practical ways in which he can help now and later on. Encourage him to take on some of the routine household tasks so you can rest. His taking responsibility for the shopping, laundry and cooking now will take the pressure off you when you first come home with your baby.

**Q.** I am worrying about writing my birth plan. I don't really know what I want!

**A.** If you write something and want to change your mind you can, even at the last moment. You do not even have to write a birth plan unless you want to. The aim of the birth plan is just to put down some notes to help the midwife when you are in labour. Think about anything that you really want to happen – or that you are really hoping to avoid. Your midwife will be able to answer any questions and will be able to write down your preferences on the notes.

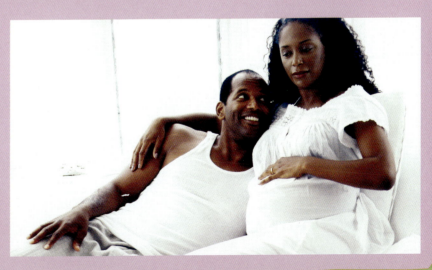

If you have a question that isn't answered here, call Tommy's pregnancy information line on **0870 777 30 60** and speak to one of our experienced midwives.

**71**

# *This is it –*
# *your baby's*

**W**hen and however you give birth, you will find it an unforgettable experience. A newborn baby makes all the waiting, worry and pain worthwhile. In this section, we look at the stages of giving birth and what might happen if your labour does not progress naturally.

If in these last few days, you start to worry about giving birth, remember that your midwives and doctors are there to support you. They are keen that this important life experience is as personal and pleasant as possible. If you have not written your birth plan, now is the time to jot some notes down and discuss them with your midwife and your birth partner. Tuck your birth plan with your notes and if you are expecting to go into labour naturally, remember to keep them with you.

You're in the last part of pregnancy, your baby's cot is ready and you've packed your hospital and baby bag. If this is your first baby, you may wonder if each twinge you feel is the start of labour.

## What does a contraction feel like?
Early contractions feel a bit like period pains. As labour progresses, the pain becomes more severe. As the muscles of the uterus contract, the pain is intense. As they relax, the pain fades.

### Fact File

A few weeks before birth, the pressure of your baby's head (or bottom, if your baby is breech) on your cervix signals your body to produce a hormone called oxytocin. This hormone makes your uterus muscles contract or tighten. As it contracts, your uterus pushes your baby down. Meanwhile, your cervix is softening and dilating (opening) to make more space for your baby to pass through. The contractions get stronger and more frequent. This is the start of labour.

### First signs
At first, you may not be sure that this is the start of labour. It can start slowly and you may wonder if it's more Braxton Hicks contractions (see page 62) or just pregnancy aches!

You are probably in labour but this can happen a few days before the start of labour and some women don't notice the show at all.

### *Top tip*

Have a clock or watch, and a notepad and pen, so you can time your contractions and write down the timings.

This is it –
Your baby's
big day!

# big day!

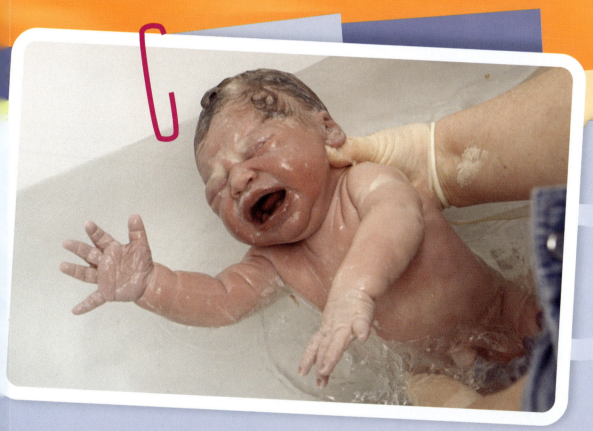

**left** Your precious
newborn baby will
make the nine
months of waiting
all worthwhile.

## Is this really it?

Labour is different for every woman and every birth and it can start so slowly that you may not be sure that this is the real thing. Typical signs that you are in labour include:

- **Contractions that last more than 40 seconds.**
- **Three contractions every 10 minutes over an hour or so.**
- **Your waters have broken – you feel a gush or trickle of liquid.**

For most women, waters break after labour contractions have started. For some women, waters break before labour starts. It's a sign that labour will start shortly!

If your waters break before labour contractions begin, phone your hospital or midwife, as there is a risk of infection. Your midwife will probably

73

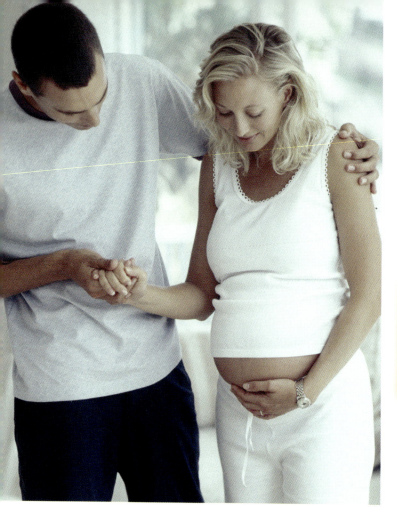

## Relax!

Labour can take a long time, and your midwife may advise you to stay at home for a while. What can you do while you wait?

- Watch TV
- Have a bath or shower
- Have a cup of tea and piece of toast – you'll need lots of energy for later
- Have a sleep (if the pain of the contractions allow!)
- Listen to some music
- Phone a friend!

*Call your midwife **immediately** if:*
- **You are losing blood**
- **The pain becomes more severe**
- **You have a severe headache**
- **You feel sick**
- **… or if you have any other worries**

## When to call your midwife or hospital

Call your midwife or the hospital whenever you feel you need to. Some women wait until their contractions are at five-minute intervals. You can always call before this time, and the hospital or midwife will tell you when to come in.

**above**   At first, you may not be sure that labour is starting.

want to see you for a check. Tell her if the waters are either smelly or coloured as this could be a sign that your baby is in distress and needs attention. If your waters are clear, you will probably be able to go home when you have been checked and given a time for labour to be induced (started artificially, see page 82) if it doesn't start naturally within 24–36 hours.

*Labour has started – what next?*

1. **Phone your partner or friend to let them know.**
2. **Time and write down the timings of contractions.**
3. **If you are unsure about when to go to hospital, phone your midwife or the hospital.**
4. **If you are having a home birth, let your midwife know that you think labour has started.**
5. **If you have other children, let your babysitter know!**
6. **Check that you have everything you need – hospital and baby bag, car keys or taxi number (and money to pay for the taxi).**
7. **Try to relax!**

all morning - period-like pains.
12noon - diarrhoea
3.05pm - first twinge? Contraction?
3.49pm - contraction? Sharp pain
4.28pm - contraction 15 seconds long
4.38pm - contraction 10 seconds - called Dave at work
  - on his way (fast!)
5.10pm - contraction 12 seconds
5.22pm - contraction 30 seconds - OUCH!
5.30pm - Dave home - contraction 20 seconds
5.32pm - Dave calls labour ward - they say stay at home as long as I can, but I'm to go in if waters break, if I start to bleed or if it's too painful
5.36pm - have a bath. more long contractions in bath
  - every 5-10mins about 30 seconds each
Out of bath - 40 seconds contraction - OUCH! and waters break!
Dave calls labour ward. 6.25pm - another 40 seconds contraction - leave the house!
45 second contraction in the car, feel more fluid trickling with each contraction...
7pm - arrive at hospital, more contractions while waiting
THIS IS IT! I'M HAVING A BABY!!!

*This is it –*
*Your baby's*
*big day!*

## First checks

- When your midwife first sees you, she will:
- Check your blood pressure, pulse and temperature
- Feel your tummy to confirm your baby's size and which way round he is
- Check your baby's heartbeat – either with cardiotocograph monitor (see below) or a trumpet-like stethoscope
- Check your cervix – you will have a vaginal examination to see how far your cervix has dilated.

She will repeat these checks approximately every four hours to check on the progress of your labour.

## Who will be there?

If you're having your baby at home, your midwife will be with you all the time unless you ask her to leave you alone with your labour companion for a while.

In hospital, your midwife will try to be with you but she or he may be looking after more than one woman. There may be a student midwife working alongside your midwife. If you feel you need your midwife, call. Your birth partner can be with you all the time.

## Checking on you and baby

Your midwife can keep an eye on your baby's progress in a number of ways:

- A **cardiotocograph** (CTG) measures your baby's heartbeat and the timing of your contractions. You wear two belts round your bump. In some hospitals, you may be able to move around with the belts on.
- **Fetal blood sampling** (FBS) shows your baby's well-being more accurately. A small amount of blood is taken from your baby's scalp (through your vagina) to check her oxygen level. If this shows your baby doesn't have enough oxygen, your care team may suggest a caesarean.

---

*There are many positions you can use to help deal with the pain and stage of labour you are in. Do what feels right for you.*

- **Squat – ask your partner to hold you from behind**
- **Lean – use a wall, bed or beanbag**
- **Rock – on all fours**
- **Kneel down – and rest over a pile of pillows or a swiss ball**
- **Kneel – hold on to your birth partner**
- **Sit – lean back on to your birth partner**
- **Walk around**
- **Rest when you need to.**

*Don't worry about what it looks like. Do what feels good!*

---

## The stages of labour
Labour has three stages. Each woman is different, and the stages may not be clear, or may last for differing amounts of time.

**First stage** Contractions make the cervix dilate to about 10 centimetres across. This is usually the longest stage. For a first baby it can last between 10 and 18 hours.

**Transition** Your cervix is nearly open and the contractions can be severe.

**Second stage** This is the hard part! Your baby moves through your vagina – with a lot of pushing from you – and is delivered. It can last for 30 minutes to a couple of hours for first babies.

**Third stage** After your baby is born, the placenta will follow. There are two ways that this can happen: you can choose either to let your body push it out naturally, which may take a couple of hours and can be associated with some blood loss, or you can choose to be given a drug to help expel it. The drug is injected into your leg immediately after your baby is born, and causes the placenta to come away from the wall of your womb, allowing your midwife to gently pull it out.

Phew! It's recovery time. It's a time to hold your baby, relax, cry, laugh and know you've done it!

- A **fetal scalp electrode** (FSE) is sometimes used with the CTG machine if the belts on the tummy don't pick up the heartbeat accurately. It is done by attaching a small electrode to your baby's scalp. This is harmless, but you cannot move around with it in place.

## Move about!

During labour it is best to stay as upright as possible as gravity helps you push the baby. Lying on your back – slows things down and can be more painful.

## When you need extra help in labour

Your doctor and midwife will encourage you to give birth as naturally as possible and in your own time, but sometimes, even after a good start, labour slows right down. This gets tiring for you and may distress your baby. You may need an intervention – something you can't do for yourself – to help deliver your baby safely.

*Interventions include:*
- **Drip**
- **Ventouse or forceps**
- **Artificial rupture of membranes (ARM)**
- **Caesarean section (see page 80)**

Intervention may mean that you are less mobile and have less control over your labour.

Try not to be disappointed if you planned a drug-free, mobile birth and you end up having monitoring and forceps. You've done your best! Ask your birth partner to discuss with your midwife ways that you can deliver your baby safely and in the way you want.

## Drip

If your contractions slow down, your doctor might suggest syntocinon, a drug that encourages the uterus to contract and the cervix to open. This will be given through a needle in your hand or arm. This is called augmentation. Having labour augmented can make contractions more painful, so you might want to talk to your midwife about pain relief, such as an epidural (see page 65). Unfortunately, the drip may mean that you can't move around as much.

**Say again?** Episiotomy: Sometimes, the perineum – the skin between the vagina and the anus – tears as your baby is born. Very occasionally your midwife may suggest cutting the perineum to widen the opening. This is called an episiotomy and is done under local anaesthetic. Afterwards you will be stitched using dissolvable stitches.

**Say again?** You might have heard your doctor or midwife using the words syntocinon, syntometrine and oxytocin. Syntocinon is the drug used to help stimulate contractions if they are slowing down. Syntometrine is given as an injection after the baby is born, to help deliver the placenta. Both drugs are known as oxytocinons, which are known to stimulate muscle contractions.

## Ventouse or forceps

If the pushing stage (stage 2) is very long and your baby is under stress, your care team may advise using a suction pad (ventouse) or forceps to help your baby out. Your baby may look a bit squashed or bruised, but this will disappear within a few days. If you have a forceps delivery, you will need an episiotomy.

## Artificial rupture of membranes

If your waters haven't broken, your obstetrician may pop the amniotic sac with a thin piece of hooked plastic. This is also called amniotomy. The procedure itself is painless, but contractions afterwards may become much more painful, so it is worth discussing your pain relief before this is done.

**below** A kneeling or all-fours position helps to open your pelvis.

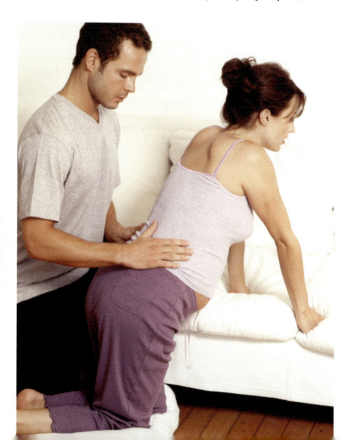

This is it –
Your baby's
big day!

# The night shift

Justina, 54, is a labour ward midwife. Here she shares her experience of the night shift.

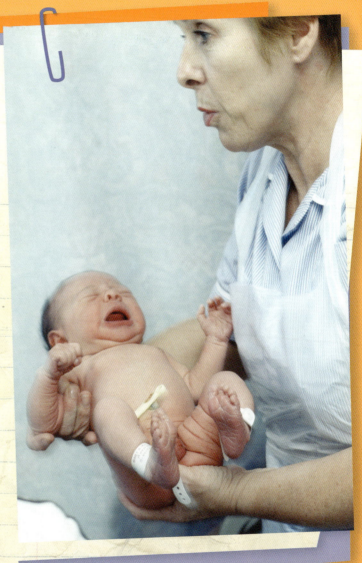

"The night shift begins at 7.00pm. For the first half an hour or so, we meet up with the day shift and they talk us through what is happening. This can take more than half an hour if there are any difficult or complicated labours in progress, but it is essential. A dayshift midwife introduces us to the woman she has been working with, so that we can take over and offer continuity. Our unit has a system where each midwife is assigned one woman to look after during her shift. This works well although when a baby is about to be delivered, we work in pairs. This means that one of us can look after the baby and the other can care for the mother.

The night shift is completely different to the day. During the day, there are doorbells ringing, visitors popping in as well as doctors and consultants coming around. At night it is calm and much less stressful, and in some ways quite special. The whole hospital is quiet and this means there is a completely different atmosphere.

At the start of a shift, you never know what will happen. Sometimes we can start off with only one woman in labour, yet at the end of the shift find ourselves with six. We always cope though because we are a small but friendly team and this makes a huge difference. Our unit is self-contained and we have an operating theatre next door, which means that if an emergency caesarean is needed, we can quickly get women ready.

We have recently been trained how to scrub up so we can help to hand the surgeon the instruments in the operating theatre. Women who are delivering twins will be taken to the operating theatre so if there is a problem in delivering the second twin, swift action can be taken. I love delivering twins – it is not always straightforward, but it is really satisfying. "

"Sometimes we can start off with only one woman in labour, yet at the end of the shift find ourselves with six. "

# First minutes of life

Well done! You may feel totally elated, exhausted, happy, amazed ... and you'll be tired, perhaps a bit shivery and probably thirsty and hungry. Time to be introduced to your baby. If you didn't know before, you will certainly know now, boy or girl!

## Hold her!

The midwife clamps and cuts the umbilical cord – this is painless for both you and your baby. You will then deliver the placenta. Your baby will be placed on your stomach or breast. If you would prefer your baby to be cleaned before she is given to you, ask your midwife (and put this in your birth plan). It's a great idea to put your baby straight to your breast to feed. You and your partner may want some minutes to share the moment quietly. Shortly after, your midwife will check your baby.

## First cries

Not all babies cry straight after the birth (although many do!) If you had a lot of pain-relieving drugs, your baby may be feeling the effect of them too and may take more time to realise the power of her lungs!

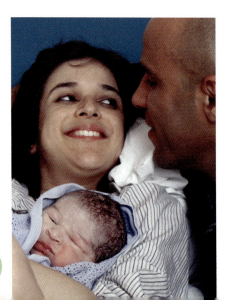

## Take a look!

Your baby may not look clean, rounded and eyes wide open. She's been on an incredibly hard journey to the outside world! Some babies have misshapen heads. Their skulls are soft and may have been moulded by the passage down a narrow birth canal. The use of forceps or ventouse (see page 76) can bruise or temporarily shape your baby's head. Don't worry – within a few days, it will change back.

## Hairy or not?

Some babies are born with a mop of hair, and others have none.

## Greasy covering

Your baby may be covered in a thick greasy layer, called the vernix that kept your baby dry while she was swimming in amniotic fluid in the uterus. If your baby is premature, she may have a thick covering of vernix, but overdue babies will have little or none.

## Fontanelles

The top of your baby's head may be pulsing. This is one of her fontanelles, where the bones of her skull have not yet fused together. It will be about a year before these bones close up.

**left** If all has gone well, your midwife will leave you and your partner to have some quiet time getting to know your new baby.

## Swollen body

Don't be surprised if your baby has slightly swollen breasts, even boys. This is to do with the pregnancy hormones. The swelling soon passes. Boys may have swollen scrotums and girls may have swollen genitals – again, the swelling will disappear.

## Belly button

You won't see your baby's belly button for a week or so. A clamp is put on a small piece of the cord to prevent bleeding. Your midwife and health visitor will show you how to clean around this, and will check it when they visit you. It will fall off naturally, revealing your baby's belly button.

## Rashes and spots

Babies are often red, spotty and rashy! Your postnatal care team (midwife and health visitor) will check any rashes, but most disappear quickly. If your baby seems unwell, and has a rash, let your doctor know as soon as possible.

## Birth marks

Your baby may have a red splodge on her face or body. Marks are common and most usually fade in time.

## First poo!

The first poo is dark green and black. It's a substance called meconium and it's the waste matter left over from the amniotic fluid your baby drank in the uterus. Over the next few days, your

**This is it –**
*Your baby's
big day!*

baby's poo will change to a green then yellow colour if breastfed, often with 'bits' in that look like seeds, and a lighter brown colour if bottlefed.

## Is my baby all right?

Your midwife will check that your baby looks OK and has all her fingers and toes. She will record your baby's condition using a system called the AGPAR scale at one minute, five minutes and sometimes ten minutes.

A total score of less than 7 on the second or last check means your baby needs medical attention and may need special care for a time. She will be seen immediately by a paediatrician (a doctor who specialises in the health of children).

### Further checks

*Your midwife will also:*
- **Weigh your baby**
- **Check your baby's spine to check for spina bifida**
- **Check mouth for cleft palate**
- **Check there are the right number of fingers and toes**
- **Measure her head**
- **Check her fontanelles**
- **Check her hips and limbs for movement**

## Going home

Your baby will need to wee, poo and feed before you can both leave hospital. It's a good idea to jot down the times of the above so you can tell your midwife when she asks – and it's easy to forget in all the activity that surrounds your newborn. A paediatrician will see your baby before she leaves hospital. You will also need to be well, not bleeding too much.

If you have a home birth, your midwife will stay with you until about two hours after the birth. After this, your midwife and then your health visitor will regularly visit.

After a straightforward birth, you can go home after a few hours, if you feel well and as long as your baby has had a wee, a poo, and a feed. Many women choose to recover their strength with a stay of one or two nights in hospital.

After a caesarean section you may need to stay in hospital for 3–5 days. When you are home, your midwife and health visitor will continue to check on you and your baby.

### First injections

You will be asked if you want your baby to have the following tests and injections:

- **Vitamin K injection or oral drops – recommended at birth as newborns often have low levels of vitamin K, which helps prevent blood clotting**
- **A heel prick blood test to check that your baby does not suffer from a thyroid deficiency, a condition called phenylketonuria, sickle-cell anaemia or thalassaemia.**
- **Hepatitis B vaccine – this is offered if you or your partner has a history of hepatitis B (see page 40).**

*Did you know?*

Many babies lose weight for the first few days. She will start to gain weight in around a week's time.

## How do you feel?

Apart from feeling emotionally elated or drained, your body may feel very sore and tired!

You may be worried about going to the loo, as urine can sting, and in case you tear any stitches. This is very unlikely – drink plenty of water and go as soon as you have the urge. Other common symptoms include:
- Leaking urine
- Cramp-like pains in your tummy
- Sweating
- Bleeding like a period.

All of these are perfectly natural. Talk to your midwife if you have any worries.

It's unusual to have complications after the birth, but if you experience the following, let your midwife know (if you are in hospital) or contact your doctor or midwife:
- Prolonged, heavy, bright red bleeding (it will be bright red for a few days and then pinky brown – contact your doctor if it turns bright red again)
- A lot of clots (or very large clots) in any bleeding
- Smelly discharge
- Pain or swelling in your calf or leg (this could be a sign of a blood clot)
- Continuous high temperature.

## Postnatal care

Care after your baby is born is called postnatal care. This continues for both you and your newborn. You'll be visited at home by your community midwife and then by your health visitor. They are always ready to listen if you have any worries about your or your baby's health.

**Say again?** **Thyroid deficiency** The thyroid is the gland that determines the rate at which the body works.

# Caesarean section

Some women need a caesarean section to give birth. This might be because your baby is in an awkward position for a vaginal birth or there are medical issues that make it necessary. An obstetrician makes a cut in your abdomen and gently lifts your baby out through it.

If you know before you go into labour that you need a caesarean section, it is called a 'planned' or 'elective' caesarean. If you had not planned one, and are in labour, you and your care team may decide this is the safest course of action – this is called an 'emergency' caesarean. This doesn't necessarily mean that you or your baby are in serious danger, just that it has not been planned.

**What happens:**
- **You will be asked lots of questions and asked to sign a consent form for the operation.**
- **You will be taken to the operating theatre**
- **The top part of your pubic hair is shaved**
- **You are given some medicine to settle your stomach**
- **A drip is put in your arm**
- **An anaesthetist gives you a regional anaesthetic**

**Say again?** A regional anaesthetic is pain relief that numbs your pelvic area but doesn't send you off to sleep, so that you can see and hear your baby being born. Regional anaesthetics include epidural (see page 65) and spinal block.

There will be quite a lot going on in the operating theatre. Your partner can be there too. As for any operation, everyone will wear surgical masks.

You can't see the operation, as a screen is put over your tummy, but you may hear many instruments. A small cut is made along the top of your bikini line and your baby is lifted out. The placenta is removed and when this third stage is complete, you are stitched, and your partner can hold your baby. The whole operation takes about an hour.

## Feelings about a caesarean

Many women feel disappointed that they will not be able to have a vaginal birth. But if you are prepared for the possibility of a caesarean, it may not seem so daunting. Having a caesarean section shouldn't delay or prevent bonding with your baby. Some mothers actually prefer caesarean section to going into labour.

**" I'll never be able to give birth 'naturally' now. "**

Many women are able to have another baby vaginally after a caesarean. This is called VBAC (vaginal birth after caesarean) and you may need some special care while you are in labour, but you should be able to deliver normally.

*Some of the main reasons you might be offered a caesarean section include:*
- **Placenta praevia (see page 59)**
- **Baby is in distress**
- **Baby is breech or another difficult position**
- **Baby is very large**

**below** A caesarean shouldn't delay or prevent you bonding with your baby.

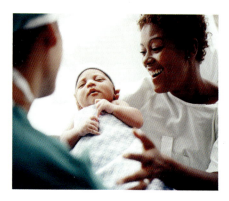

## Recovery

It takes time to recover from a caesarean section, and you will need to stay in hospital for about 3–5 days. Your stitches need to heal and you may need strong painkillers. You may be on a drip for a while. You can still breastfeed and hold your baby.

You usually have internal stitches which dissolve on their own and one stitch on the outside that your community midwife can remove around the fifth day after your operation.

This is it –
Your baby's
big day!

# Babies who arrive early

There is usually little warning that a baby is going to come early. If you go into labour prematurely, the antenatal team will keep close checks on your baby and will most likely take him for checks as soon as he is born.

## Causes

Some causes of premature labour include:
- **Waters breaking early**
- **Placenta is not functioning properly**
- **Pre-eclampsia**
- **Twins or more**
- **Infection**

The labour is usually shorter as your baby is smaller than a full-term baby.

## Signs

If you experience any of the following before your baby is due, contact your midwife, doctor or hospital as soon as possible:
- **Cramps like period pains, sometimes with diarrhoea or vomiting**
- **Pink or brown vaginal discharge**
- **Waters breaking**
- **Lower backache or pressure**
- **Contractions**

If your antenatal team can delay premature labour they will try, because usually the longer your baby is in your body, the better his health.

## What happens to your baby

If your baby is born prematurely, he will need special care for a while. Babies born before around 34 weeks of pregnancy are likely to be put in the special care baby unit while their bodies mature and develop. Babies born after 32 weeks may be able to breastfeed or feed from a bottle. Before this time, they will often need to be fed by tube.

In SCBU, your baby will be put in an incubator to control his:
- **Breathing – he can be given oxygen if necessary**
- **Temperature – he can't sweat so he needs to be kept at an even temperature**
- **Feeding – he can be fed through a tube in his nose.**

**Say again?** Pronounced 'skerboo', SCBU stands for Special Care Baby Unit, and it is where premature babies are first cared for. Babies who need more intensive care may be transferred to NICU, a neonatal intensive care unit – which may be at another hospital.

You will be encouraged to look at your baby, talk to him and when possible hold him. It's especially important for premature babies to have breastmilk so your midwife will encourage you to express milk regularly which can then be given to your baby. This means your breastmilk will be plentiful when your baby is able to drink from the breast.

### "I want to hold my baby"

It may not always be possible to hold your baby straightaway if she is premature. This can feel incredibly disappointing but you will be able to hold her as soon as possible.

### How long does a premature baby stay in hospital?

Premature babies often need to stay in hospital until the time they were originally due. They will need to be gaining weight and breathing independently (although they may need some extra oxygen) before leaving special care.

# Babies who arrive late

$S$ome babies get so comfortable in there that they don't seem in any hurry to come out! You may need a little bit of extra help to get labour started – this is called induction.

## When is a baby overdue?

Only one baby in five is born by their due date, so try to relax if you pass the due date. However, when your baby has gone around seven days past her due date your healthcare team will begin to monitor. After a while the placenta begins to age, which means she may not be receiving enough oxygen and nutrients. You can choose not to be induced straight away, but your care team will advise you if it's necessary for the health of your baby.

## Membrane sweep

You may be offered a membrane sweep. This involves a vaginal examination – using her finger, the midwife 'sweeps' the cervix and tries to stimulate contractions. If this doesn't work, you may be offered a date for induction. Induction is a way of kick-starting your body into labour when your baby is overdue.

**Say again?** A pessary is a small tablet that administers medication through the vagina.

## How will my baby be induced?

Your midwife inserts a gel or pessary into your vagina. This contains a drug called prostaglandin that helps to open the cervix enough for your waters to be broken. This method can take a while, and doesn't always work.

You may also be offered a syntocinon drip (see page 76).

**Did you know?**

If you are overdue, or want to try natural ways to start labour, some women suggest:
- raspberry leaf tea (it is very important that you don't drink this before 37 weeks in case it sends you into premature labour)
- sex – your partner's semen contains natural prostaglandins that stimulate labour
- a hot curry
- stimulating your nipples

You may even find that just setting a date for induction sends you into natural labour!

Don't listen to anyone who tells you that castor oil will do the trick – it will just give you horrible diarrhoea and stomach cramps that aren't labour pains.

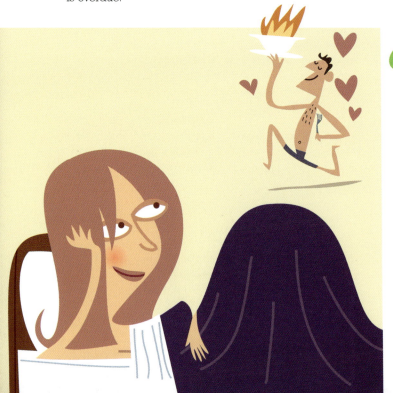

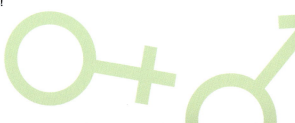

**left** If you can face them, a hot curry and/or sex with your partner can help!

This is it –
Your baby's
big day!

# More questions about birth

## Q&A

**Q.** I'm worried that I will not know when my labour has started.

**A.** This is a common worry for first-time mothers, although once labour gets really under way, you will definitely know. You may find that your waters break, in which case you know that labour is, or soon will be, under way, or you may start by feeling contractions. These contractions differ from the practice contractions known as Braxton Hicks that you may already have had. They feel stronger, deeper and more painful. Look out too for waves of backache as some women find that this is where they feel the contractions.

Once labour is established, contractions become more regular and are not going away! When you are having contractions every five or ten minutes, think about either going into hospital or, if you have a chosen a home birth, contacting your midwife.

If you don't know whether you're in labour, telephone the labour ward or the midwife who is looking after you. They are used to dealing with false alerts so don't worry.

**Q.** I'm finding it hard to sleep because I keep on worrying about the birth. I can't see how I will manage.

**A.** Giving birth often feels daunting, especially if other women have been telling you about their experiences. It is worth remembering that you are not going to be facing this alone. You will have a midwife who will be there to support and help you. Her experience and knowledge will mean that you'll be guided through the birth. She'll also offer you pain relief.

Talk to your midwife now about how you're feeling so you can talk through your choices. Think too about things that you might like to have around you during labour that will help you to relax. This might mean music, candles or a favourite perfume.

Most women want someone they know well with them to act as a birth partner. This can be a friend, relative or partner. Choose someone who you trust and will be good at keeping you company.

**Q.** My partner insists that he wants to cut the umbilical cord. Is this possible?

**A.** Some midwives automatically offer partners the opportunity to cut the umbilical cord when your baby is born. If you want this, put it in your birth plan and remind your midwife during the birth. There are times when this will not be possible, for example, if either you or your baby are in need of attention. Your partner needs to be ready to see how everything goes on the day.

**Q.** My friend said that she got depressed after giving birth. Can this really happen?

**A.** In the first five days, many women find that they experience a rollercoaster of emotions. As well as amazing feelings of happiness and joy, some women also find that they suddenly become tearful and quite depressed. This is very common on day three or four and is even known as the 'baby blues'. Changing hormones cause these feelings. Exhaustion and the realisation of the responsibility can also play a part.

For most women, this quickly passes and feelings of happiness soon return. A few women get a longer type of depression known as postnatal depression. If you do find that you're not enjoying your baby, don't be afraid of telling someone. Your midwife, doctor or health visitor will be ready to listen and support you. Postnatal depression is not something to feel ashamed of, and there are support networks (see page 106) to help you cope. It is not a sign that you'll be a bad mother.

If you have a question that isn't answered here, call Tommy's pregnancy information line on **0870 777 30 60** and speak to one of our experienced midwives.

83

# Happy &

You might be starting to think about how being pregnant will affect your daily life. This section looks at ways in which you can keep fit and healthy, and looks at other areas of your life such as relationships, work and money. It also includes an article about having twins and multiple births. Men can be brilliant at helping during pregnancy and can make fantastic birth partners. Knowing how important they can be, we've written a few pages just for them.

## Fit and healthy

If you are sociable and you like your food, being pregnant shouldn't stop you from having fun. Some foods are better than others. Something from everything you eat, drink or smoke crosses the placenta to your baby. So the better you look after yourself, the better start you give your baby.

You don't need a special diet – and you certainly don't need to 'eat for two' – but you do need to get a balance of foods. Make sure you're eating foods from each of the groups shown in the table opposite every day.

## Extras

**Folic acid:** Folic acid helps in the early formation of the baby's nervous system. Lack of folic acid can cause spina bifida, where the baby's spine doesn't close up properly. Broccoli, sprouts, spinach and other green leafy vegetables, and nuts, all contain folic acid, but doctors still recommend a supplement – 400 mcg a day in the first 12 weeks of pregnancy. Even better, start taking it before you conceive.

**Essential fatty acids:** These help your baby's brain to develop, and may make for an easier pregnancy. You can find these in nuts and seeds, lean meat and 'oily' fish such as salmon or mackerel. It's not advisable to eat more than two portions of oily fish a week.

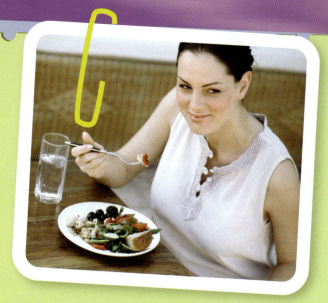

**above**  You should only 'eat for one' with a healthy balance of foods.

*Take care out and about*
- **Carry your notes with you everywhere.**
- **On public transport, book seats in advance if you can. If not, be ready to ask for a seat if you need to.**
- **Pace yourself so you don't get overtired, especially in hot weather.**
- **After 28 weeks, check before you book air tickets that the airline will accept you.**
- **Wash your hands before you eat.**

# healthy

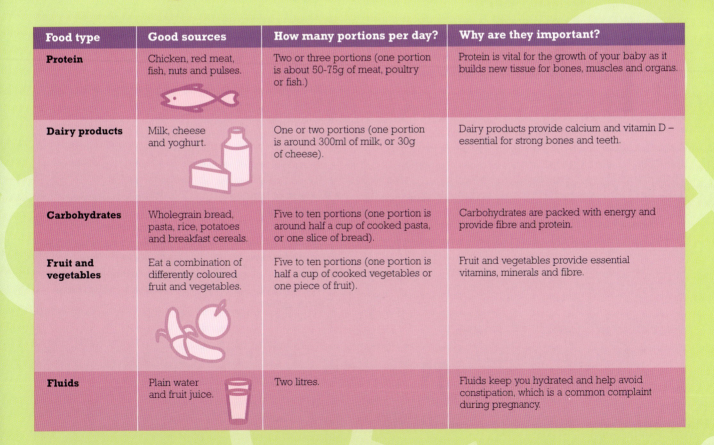

| Food type | Good sources | How many portions per day? | Why are they important? |
|---|---|---|---|
| **Protein** | Chicken, red meat, fish, nuts and pulses. | Two or three portions (one portion is about 50-75g of meat, poultry or fish.) | Protein is vital for the growth of your baby as it builds new tissue for bones, muscles and organs. |
| **Dairy products** | Milk, cheese and yoghurt. | One or two portions (one portion is around 300ml of milk, or 30g of cheese). | Dairy products provide calcium and vitamin D – essential for strong bones and teeth. |
| **Carbohydrates** | Wholegrain bread, pasta, rice, potatoes and breakfast cereals. | Five to ten portions (one portion is around half a cup of cooked pasta, or one slice of bread). | Carbohydrates are packed with energy and provide fibre and protein. |
| **Fruit and vegetables** | Eat a combination of differently coloured fruit and vegetables. | Five to ten portions (one portion is half a cup of cooked vegetables or one piece of fruit). | Fruit and vegetables provide essential vitamins, minerals and fibre. |
| **Fluids** | Plain water and fruit juice. | Two litres. | Fluids keep you hydrated and help avoid constipation, which is a common complaint during pregnancy. |

# Piling on the pounds

Linda, 24, shows how easy it is to pile on the pounds when you are pregnant – and how difficult to lose them afterwards.

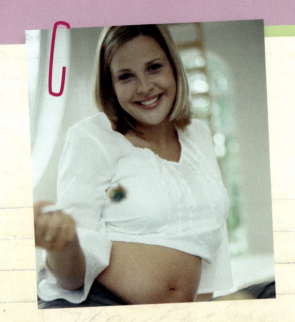

**above** Power snacks will help you back into shape after your baby is born.

"I've always been a bit on the plump side, but when I found out that I was pregnant, it was like an excuse to eat more. The more I grew, the more I ate as it didn't seem to matter any more. I really regret that now as, had I held back a bit, I think I would have lost the weight more easily. The turning point came after Rhia was a year old and I caught sight of myself in a shop window.

That was it and I was lucky because my doctor's practice gave me a lot of support and good advice about food. I am better at buying the right food now and bit by bit the weight slipped off. It's great because I am slimmer now than I was before I fell pregnant.

*I caught sight of myself in a shop window. That was it.*

## Don't pig out!

These foods won't harm your baby, but like Linda, you'll find they will pile on the pounds because of their high fat or sugar content, and you'll find it hard to shift the weight after your baby is born. So – treats only!

- Butter and margarine
- Oil-based dressings, including mayonnaise
- Cream
- Crisps and chips
- Fried food
- Burgers
- Pizza
- Pastry
- Ice cream
- Chocolate and sweets
- Biscuits
- Cakes
- Puddings

## Gaining weight

There is no average weight gain in pregnancy as every woman is different. This is why you are not likely to be weighed at each antenatal visit. Most pregnant women have an increased appetite at times, so if you are extra hungry, choose from our list of **healthy** snacks.

## Power snacks

- Packets of raisins
- Carrot sticks
- Celery sticks
- Low-fat yoghurt
- Dried apricots
- Satsumas
- Sliced melon
- Sliced apple
- Cherry tomatoes
- Hummus and breadsticks
- Baked beans on toast
- Vegetable soups
- Vegetable sticks and low-fat yoghurt dip

# Foods to avoid

## Foods that may cause infection or illness

| Infection | Caused by | Symptoms (if any) | Effects on baby | Foods to avoid |
|---|---|---|---|---|
| **Listeria** | A bacterium called Listeria. | Mild gastroenteritis or flu-like illness. | Can lead to miscarriage and stillbirth. | Pâté (including vegetarian), unpasteurised dairy products and mould ripened cheeses (e.g. Brie, Camembert) and blue cheeses (e.g. Stilton). Cheese made from pasteurised milk is fine, including hard or creamed cheese, mozzarella, ricotta or yogurt). Ready-cooked meals may contain Listeria, so heat thoroughly. |
| **Salmonella** | A bacterium called Salmonella, which is a common cause of food poisoning. | Vomiting, abdominal pain, diarrhoea and nausea. | Can lead to miscarriage and stillbirth. | Raw eggs or undercooked meat can contain Salmonella. Cook eggs thoroughly so that whites and yolk are solid. Mayonnaise mousses and meringues may contain raw egg. Shop-bought non-refrigerated mayonnaise is safe. |
| **Toxoplasmosis** | A tiny parasite that lives in cat poo and in raw meat. | Mother may not notice any symptoms. | Miscarriage, brain damage, blindness. | Avoid raw or undercooked meat and smoked-only or cured meat like Parma ham. Avoid unwashed vegetables and fruit, and unpasteurised goat's milk products. Wear gloves when handling cat litter and gardening. |

## Other foods to avoid

**Liver and liver sausage:** Love it or hate it, liver is off the menu when you are pregnant. Liver contains too much vitamin A and it can harm the baby.

**Peanuts and shellfish:** If you have a family history of eczema or asthma or allergies to peanuts, dairy products or shellfish, avoid any foods that trigger your allergy while you are pregnant and breastfeeding. This gives your baby the best chance of not developing the allergy later on. Raw shellfish should always be avoided in pregnancy.

**Caffeine:** This is found not only in coffee and tea, but also in colas and some 'power' drinks: Stick to two cups a day as caffeine can dehydrate you, stop your body from taking up iron and may cause miscarriage.

## Food poisoning

Food poisoning is common, and can be nasty if you are pregnant and can put your baby's health at risk. You can take simple steps to prevent it.

✓ **Wash your hands before handling food**
✓ **Keep pets away from your food**
✓ **Keep food covered and if perishable stored in the fridge**
✓ **Separate raw and cooked food in your fridge – put raw food at the bottom to stop it dripping on to cooked food.**
✓ **Wash fruit and vegetables**
✓ **Cook meat, poultry and fish thoroughly**
✓ **Prepare raw meat, fish and poultry using different boards and knives from the ones you use to prepare vegetables**
✓ **Reheat any food until it is absolutely piping hot – and only reheat it once**
✓ **Read manufacturer's instructions when cooking ready meals**
✓ **Allow food to defrost completely, unless following manufacturer's instructions**
✓ **Keep an eye on the 'use before' date**
✓ **Check the temperature of your fridge**
✓ **If you're at a wedding or christening buffet, don't nibble on food that's been around for a few hours. Bacteria multiply very quickly!**

## Alcohol and you

Fun does not have to stop when you're pregnant, but there are a few things you'll need to cut down on or even cut out for a while. Alcohol is one of them as it can affect the healthy growth of your baby.

### Safe limits

Heavy drinking can really harm the baby, and it isn't certain exactly how much is a safe amount to drink. Some women prefer not to drink at all, especially in the first three months of pregnancy when the baby's development is still in the early stages. If you enjoy a drink, try to keep to around two units a week. Do not binge drink or drink enough to be drunk. Remember that your baby feels the effects, too!

### What is a unit of alcohol?

Most people serve themselves generous glasses at home without measuring them! One unit is approximately:

- **25ml pub measure of spirits such as vodka, gin or rum**
- **125ml glass of wine**
- **¼ pint of 'extra strong' beer, lager or cider**
- **½ pint of ordinary strength beer, lager or cider**

Some drinks are stronger than others – if you want to work out your units more accurately there is an alcohol units calculator on www.portmangroup.org.uk.

*Try these:*
- **Fruit smoothies**
- **Iced fruit teas (but not raspberry leaf tea)**
- **Traditional still lemonade**
- **Milk shakes – use skimmed milk**
- **Yoghurt drinks – look for low-fat yoghurt**
- **And for something special – orange sunset – grenadine syrup with pineapple juice and orange juice**

### *Top tip*

- Ask for low-alcohol or alcohol-free drinks.
- Avoid eating salty snacks such as nuts and crisps with alcohol. These will make you feel more thirsty, so you will drink more quickly!
- Have a glass of water before the alcoholic drink so you are not so thirsty.
- Add extra mixers such as lemonade and tonic to make drinks last longer.

## Q&A

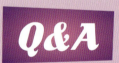

Take time to enjoy your food, and do not skip meals.

**Q.** I'm overweight. Can I diet while I am pregnant?

**A.** If by diet you mean a weight loss programme that cuts out vital nutrients, then no. But if you mean 'making healthy changes' – as many diets do now – you'll feel great and give your baby a better chance. Replace cakes, crisps, biscuits and sweets with plenty of fresh fruit and vegetables – and drink plenty of water.

**Q.** Should I take iron tablets?

**A.** No, not unless your doctor has prescribed them for you. You can get all the iron you need from your food as long as you haven't got particularly low levels of iron. Eat plenty of red meat and dark green vegetables and wholemeal bread and fortified breakfast cereals. The body takes iron more easily when foods that contain vitamin C are

present. If you start the day with a glass of orange juice and wholemeal toast or fortified cereals you'll be well on your way. Tell your midwife if you are vegetarian – she'll advise you on the best way to keep your iron levels up.

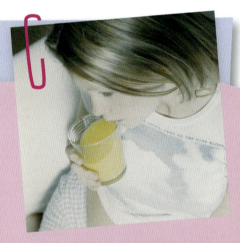

# Drugs, tablets & pills

**P**regnancy is a time to think about what you are putting into your body. The chemicals in some drugs can affect the growing baby even though normally they may not have any side effects. It's best not to take any over-the-counter medicines without checking with your pharmacist first. If you have been taking medication, check with your doctor that it is still safe to use. You should also try to stop using any recreational drugs such as ecstasy, cannabis or cocaine, and ask for help if you find it difficult to give these up.

## Q&A

**Q.** Can I take a paracetamol if I get a headache?

**A.** Plain paracetamol is usually fine as long as you keep to the recommended dose. Aspirin and ibuprofen are not recommended in pregnancy.

It's much better to think about why you have the headache in the first place, and try to sort it out in another way. Maybe you are tired, stressed or dehydrated. Can you take a nap, a break or drink more water? If you have severe or persistent headaches, tell your midwife – and seek help straight away if your vision is blurred or you see flashing lights (see pre-eclampsia, page 58).

**Q.** I have been smoking cannabis for a while. Will it harm my baby?

**A.** Cannabis is usually mixed with tobacco to smoke, so it carries the same risks to your baby as smoking cigarettes. And a rolled spliff doesn't filter tar and toxins as a tipped cigarette does. The effects of cannabis on the unborn baby are still being researched – the best advice is to stop while you are pregnant. If you find it hard to stop taking cannabis – or harder drugs – talk to your doctor or midwife. They will be able to advise you and to put you in contact with special drug addiction advisers.

**Q.** Can I take herbal remedies when I am pregnant?

**A.** Complementary therapies such as herbalism are popular and many women find them helpful, but herbal medicines are chemicals, even though they come from plants. So it is important to

check with your doctor that they are safe to take, especially if you are already taking any other medication. Just because you can buy something in a chemist or health shop does not mean that it will be safe for you in pregnancy. If you are thinking about using complementary therapies it is best to see a qualified practitioner (see page 106) who will know what is and isn't safe to use in pregnancy.

**Q.** I have heard that aromatherapy can be good.

**A.** Aromas can help us to relax and so some women find them to be useful. They can also be powerful and some aren't recommended for use in pregnancy – again, you are always best using aromatherapy guided by a qualified practitioner. Some women find aromatherapy helpful during labour so, if you are interested, it is worth visiting a practitioner in plenty of time.

# Time to quit smoking

Most people know that smoking can damage your health, but what do you do if you are a smoker and are now pregnant? No-one can force you to give up smoking, but it is important to understand the risks to your growing baby. Smoking starves the baby of oxygen and so affects its growth. Smokers are more likely to have a small or premature baby. Smoking has also been linked with cot death.

## Q&A

**Q.** I want to give up smoking – what should I do?

**A.** Wanting to give up is half way there! You are ready for a quit programme and being pregnant is the best motivation you'll ever get. There is a lot of help available for people who want to give up smoking. Your doctor or midwife will be keen to support you and point you in the right direction, or see page 106 for support groups who can help you.

**Q.** Can I have nicotine patches if I am pregnant?

**A.** There are many different ways in which you can be helped to give up smoking. Talk to your doctor or midwife who will be able to look for the most suitable method. Nicotine patches are not advisable for use in pregnancy.

**Q.** I have tried to stop smoking but can't give up. Will cutting down make any difference?

**A.** The ideal is always to give up smoking completely. If you really can't, then cut down as much as you can – this can make a difference. Switch to the lowest tar you can and don't smoke right to the end of the cigarette. Smoke cigarettes with a filter, as these are less damaging than roll-ups. In the longer term, do think about how you might give up, as smoking is likely to affect your health and your baby's health as he grows up. Your midwife or doctor can put you in touch with local quit-smoking counsellors who will give you many tips and targets for cutting down.

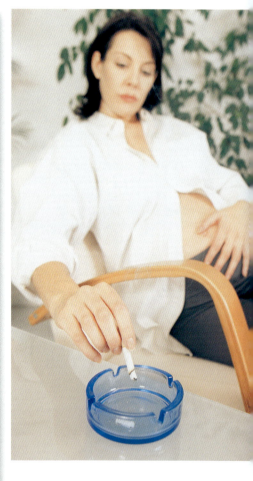

**above** Being pregnant may be just the motivation you need to quit smoking, and your midwife can support you.

# keep fit, keep moving...

Being pregnant is much harder work if you're not taking any gentle exercise. We are not talking marathons here but simply gentle walking, swimming and anything else that you enjoy. By keeping fit, you will not only feel better, but will help your baby too as you breathe in more oxygen.

## Posture

Start thinking about the way you sit and stand! Back pain is a common problem in pregnancy, especially in later months. You can prevent many problems with good posture.

## Standing

Here's an uncurling exercise to bring you up to a good standing posture. It's good to do if you have been sitting down for a long time.

- **Stand with your feet slightly apart and look down at your feet**
- **Tighten the back of your knees**
- **Tilt your pelvis forward (but don't arch your back)**
- **Point your breasts forward**
- **Bring your shoulders up to your ears, roll them back and then let them go**
- **Look up and point your chin forward**

See how much taller you feel! Try and come back to this upright posture every time you feel yourself slumping.

## Sitting

It can be tempting to crumple into a sofa or armchair after a long day, but this not good for your back. Bring your feet nearer to the chair and push your bottom well into the back of the chair

 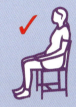

Putting your feet up helps your circulation and so helps to prevent puffy ankles and varicose veins. You can do this in a chair with your feet on a desk or table in front of you.

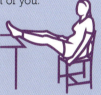

Or lie down with your feet raised on a small stool or cushion.

## Squatting

Bending from the waist to pick up anything on the floor puts a large strain on your back. Practise squatting – this will strengthen your leg muscles, which will also help you in labour. And it will be good practice for the time when your baby is a toddler and wants to be picked up, Say 'bottom to floor' when you next find yourself bending over forwards!

Standing tall, sitting well and squatting down isn't just good for pregnancy – it helps your friends, family and partner too! Try to remind each other when you see them slumped.

| Some simple steps can help your pregnancy run smoothly! | |
|---|---|
| **Rest & relaxation** | Helps to keep the blood pressure down. |
| **Basic hygiene** | Washing fruit and vegetables, wearing gloves if you garden or change cat litter – this prevents toxoplasmosis, a dangerous condition for your baby. |
| **Exercise** | Can prevent piles, constipation, varicose veins and even kidney infections. |
| **Healthy eating & drinking** | Keeps you and your baby in the best possible health. |
| **Going to antenatal appointments** | Allows your experienced healthcare team to check on you and your baby. |
| **Going to antenatal classes** | Allows you to find out more about labour and birth. |

## Keep Moving

**Walking:** Try a brisk short walk each day. Instead of taking the bus or car, try to walk instead.

**Swimming:** This is excellent all-round exercise. It is great in late pregnancy, as it will make you feel light. If you do not swim, look out for water-based exercise classes like aquafit which offer aerobic exercise without impact on your joints.

**Yoga:** This will help your body to stay supple. Find out about local classes and tell your teacher that you are pregnant.

### Already exercising?

There is no need to give up exercises and classes that you were doing before, unless your doctor or midwife says so. Exercises and sports to avoid are those where:

- **you risk hurting your tummy**
- **you could fall**
- **you put stress on your joints**

These include high-impact exercises where you come down hard on the floor, contact sports and vigorous racket sports like squash.

Tell your instructor or teacher that you are pregnant. They can recommend safe levels of exercise.

### Top tip

- Do not exercise on an empty or full stomach – have a snack or light meal an hour or so earlier.
- Drink lots of water.
- Be ready to stop if you feel tired, uncomfortable, out of breath, lightheaded or overheated.
- The best sign that you are within safe limits is the 'talk test' – if you can keep up a normal conversation while you are exercising, this is a good sign that your heart is not pounding too hard.

### Not exercising?

*If you do not normally walk or take exercise:*
- **Build up gradually**
- **Look out for yoga and aquafit classes for pregnant women**
- **Go walking with a partner or friend**

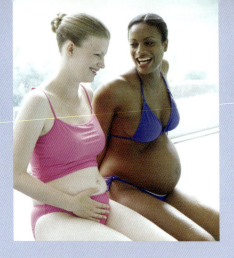

**above** Swimming is a great exercise for pregnancy.

### Keeping well at work

Most women are able to work while they are pregnant, but some jobs or tasks carry risks. They include working with chemicals, heavy lifting and manual work. Working with animals and young children may also carry a risk of picking up an infection. It's important to tell your employer you're pregnant.

Your employer has a duty to keep you safe while you are at work and they must check that your work will not affect your health. This is called risk assessment. You should also tell your GP and midwife about your work, so they can advise you. If your work is not suitable while you are pregnant, your employer must either:

- **find you alternative work at the same pay**
- **suspend you on full pay until there is no further risk to you or the baby's health.**

### Top tip

- Avoid standing for long periods – ask for a chair or stool to help you and wear support tights.
- Drink plenty of water – bring a bottle of water to work and keep it filled.
- Avoid heavy lifting – ask someone to help.
- Read and follow health and safety instructions properly – if you are not sure ask for advice.
- Tell your employer if you feel overtired or find any aspect of your work difficult.

### Top tip

Don't forget your pelvic floor exercises! (see page 9). These will help your control during labour and will also help the recovery of your vagina after the birth.

# Problems in pregnancy

$M$ost aches and pains are normal in pregnancy. But if you feel unwell, or suspect that something is not right, don't wait. Tell your doctor or midwife. It's better to be on the safe side.

## Common problems

| Problem | Caused by | What can help | When to call your doctor or midwife |
|---|---|---|---|
| **Morning sickness** | Pregnancy hormones | • Snack on ginger biscuits – even first thing in the morning!<br>• Eat small amounts regularly<br>• Drink peppermint tea<br>• Eat some day-old popcorn | If you are excessively sick and can't even keep down water, see your doctor or midwife. |
| **Backache** | Your baby's growth, weight change and relaxing muscles | • Avoid lifting<br>• Stress can make backache worse – relax as much as you can<br>• Put a hot water bottle behind your back (but not on your tummy)<br>• Check your posture | If the backache is low down and feels different, this could be a sign of premature labour. If it is severe, you may be able to see an osteopath or physiotherapist. |
| **Varicose veins** | Extra weight, increase of hormones, and increased blood flow | • Avoid standing for long periods<br>• Don't cross your legs – it slows down the blood flow<br>• Gently stretch and flex your feet<br>• Wear support tights<br>• Wear low, comfortable shoes | Check the symptoms (including pain in the legs, swollen visible veins and itchiness) with your doctor to make sure there is no inflammation or blood clotting. |
| **Piles** | Pressure on blood vessels and pregnancy hormones | • Drink plenty of water<br>• Take regular exercise<br>• Eat fibre-rich foods | If they become too uncomfortable or if there is any bleeding. |
| **Constipation** | Relaxing muscles slow down your bowel | • Drink plenty of water (aim for six to eight glasses a day)<br>• Eat plenty of fibre-rich foods such as fruit and vegetables in your diet (see page 85)<br>• Exercise regularly (see page 91) | If this doesn't help. |
| **Heartburn** (a burning sensation in your chest) | The relaxing effect of hormones allows stomach acids to rise. | • Eat small meals<br>• Avoid spicy or fatty fried foods | If it is very bad, your doctor or midwife may suggest a medicine that is suitable for use in pregnancy. |
| **Dizziness and fainting** | Your baby makes an extra demand on your body's blood supply | • If you feel light-headed, sit down and slowly put your head between your knees<br>• To prevent dizziness, eat regularly and keep your fluid intake up. Avoid getting up too quickly | If you faint, tell your midwife or doctor as soon as possible. Tell him or her about the dizziness at the next check-up. |

| Problem | Caused by | What can help | When to call your doctor or midwife |
|---|---|---|---|
| **Leg Cramps** (sharp knot of pain in your leg or foot) | Extra weight causes your muscles to tire more easily | • Firmly massage the area to try and lessen the pain<br>• Gently stretch and flex your feet and legs | If you suffer persistently, check with your doctor that there is no blood clot, a sign of thrombosis. |
| **Puffy ankles and wrists** | Increased fluids in your body | • Put your feet up whenever you can<br>• Avoid tight-fitting socks or shoes<br>• Loosen your watch strap and take off your rings if they feel uncomfortable | If you have other symptoms such as swelling in your face, a headache, blurred vision, increased blood pressure or a sudden unexplained weight gain, contact your GP or midwife as soon as possible as this may be a sign of pre-eclampsia. |
| **Carpal tunnel syndrome** (pain and numbness in some of your fingers) | If you do get puffy wrists this may compress a nerve causing a tingly sensation in your fingers | • Shake your hands and take a break from what you are doing<br>• If you use a keyboard, press lightly, keeping your elbows higher than your wrist<br>• Use your whole hand if you are lifting an object | Talk to your doctor if the symptoms persist as you can see a physiotherapist for some helpful exercises. |
| **Thrush** (vaginal itchiness and often with a smelly white discharge) | Bugs usually found in the vagina multiply too fast. | • Avoid wearing tight trousers or pants<br>• Ask the pharmacist for some cream (tell him/her you are pregnant) | Tell your doctor or midwife that you have thrush. |
| **Urinary infections such as cystitis** (feeling the need to wee more often and a burning sensation when you do so) | Due to bladder muscles relaxing and more open to infection | • Drink plenty of water and cranberry juice that helps flush out the bacteria that cause infection<br>• Fully empty your bladder when you wee | See your doctor as you may need antibiotics. Untreated infections can lead to premature labour. |
| **Feeling hot** | The speed at which your body works (your metabolic rate) increases in pregnancy | • Drink plenty (not including coffee, tea or fizzy drinks)<br>• Rest when you need to<br>• Wear cotton or natural fibres | If you have a temperature above 37.5° C. |
| **Bleeding gums and increased plaque** | Due to hormonal changes | • Cut back on sweets and chocolates – snack on fruit, crackers or nuts (unless you or someone in your family has an allergy)<br>• Carry with you a spare toothbrush and toothpaste so you can brush your teeth after meals<br>• Chew sugarless gum or have a piece of cheese after your meal to prevent dental decay | Have at least one check-up with your dentist – tell the dentist you are pregnant as X-rays are not advisable in pregnancy. |
| **Nosebleeds** | Due to pregnancy hormones | • Pinch the bridge of your nose and lean forward slightly | If the bleeding is heavy and frequent. |
| **Leaking wee** | Pressure of baby on bladder | • Drink plenty of fluids<br>• Wear a light pad<br>• Practise your pelvic floor exercises (see page 9) | If leaking is prolonged, discoloured or a gush, see your doctor or go to the hospital as your waters may have broken early (see page 72). |

## Urgent symptoms

If you experience any of the following, call your doctor or midwife straight away. If you can't get through to them, phone your hospital and they will advise you what to do. If you feel very unwell, ask someone to take you to hospital.

- **Vaginal bleeding**
- **Severe vomiting in a short time**
- **Severe itching in the last few months of pregnancy, especially on your feet or hands**
- **Severe tummy pain**
- **Signs of premature labour (see page 81)**
- **Severe persistent headache (especially from week 13 onwards)**
- **Not having a wee in 24 hours even though you are drinking**
- **Not feeling your baby move 10 times in a day from week 30 (see page 36)**
- **Sudden swelling of hands, fingers, face or ankles**
- **Blurring of vision, seeing double or seeing flashing lights**
- **A temperature higher than 37.5°C**
- **Swollen or red leg**

If your doctor has diagnosed a particular condition, follow the advice of your antenatal care team. If you have Group B Streptococcus, go to hospital at the start of labour so you can be given antibiotics.

**Say again?** Group B Streptococcus is a bacterial infection that damages red blood cells and threatens a newborn baby's ability to fight infections. Antibiotic treatment for the mother is vital to reduce the baby's risk of catching this infection.

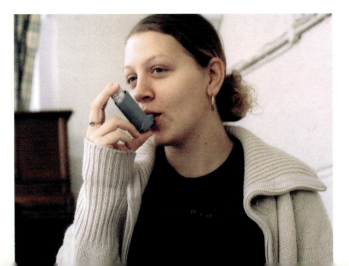

## Existing medical conditions

Usually, there is no reason that an existing medical condition should prevent you from having a happy, healthy pregnancy. You'll need to tell your doctor and midwife about any changes in your condition. And you may need more antenatal appointments than other women – make sure you keep them.

**Anaemia:** You may need iron supplements during your pregnancy.

**Depression.** If you suffer from depression and take antidepressants, check with your doctor that they are suitable for use in pregnancy. If you feel very low and the mood doesn't lift, talk to your doctor or midwife. Don't be ashamed about your feelings – many women have them. Don't bottle them up. You may need some counselling or other support, or antidepressants (suitable for use in pregnancy) for a while.

**Diabetes:** If you are already diabetic or develop diabetes in pregnancy (gestational diabetes), you will probably have more check-ups than other women. Make sure you follow medical advice about diet and exercise – and take plenty of rest.

**Asthma:** Keep your inhaler or medication with you always (but only use medication prescribed for use in pregnancy). Sometimes asthma can become more troublesome in pregnancy and labour.

**Epilepsy:** Some women with epilepsy experience more seizures in pregnancy – others do not. Your doctor or midwife may refer you to a specialist who will monitor how your epilepsy affects your pregnancy, and discuss possible changes to your treatment.

**High blood pressure:** You will need as much rest and relaxation as possible. You may need to start maternity leave early. Tell your doctor or midwife if you experience any blurred vision, swelling or headaches. Your blood pressure will also be monitored regularly and you may need to take medication to stabilise it.

**Physical disabilities:** You probably know your body and your capabilities better than anyone! Tell your midwife about your requirements. If you have a spinal injury, you may be more vulnerable to kidney and bladder problems, anaemia and muscle spasms. Attend all your appointments, rest when you can, follow a healthy diet and drink plenty of water.

**left** Ask your doctor if you need to change your asthma medication while you are pregnant.

# Feelings & relationships

**P**regnancy can be a testing time – nine months full of emotions, hormones and fear of the unknown. Here are some of the common emotions women and their partners face.

## Q&A

**Q.** I am nearly three months pregnant and feel depressed, even though it was me that wanted this baby in the first place.

**A.** The first three months of pregnancy can be rough. You're about to make a huge life change and part of you needs time to take this in. Physically, you're also likely to be tired and affected by mood-changing hormones. You will probably feel very different in a few weeks' time, but you shouldn't have to cope alone. Talk to your midwife or doctor about how you're feeling, so they can help you. And take time to talk to your partner. A little honesty can help you both to explore your feelings. It may be that your partner doesn't know how you are feeling and so isn't giving you as much support as you need.

**right** If pregnancy is getting you down, try to talk – to your partner, your doctor, your midwife – or call the trained midwives on Tommy's pregnancy information line 0870 777 30 60.

**Q.** I had a lot of difficulties in getting pregnant and in the end had two cycles of IVF. My midwife is nice, but says that unless there are any complications, I will only have the usual scans and tests. I feel that no one is interested in me any more.

**A.** IVF and other methods of assisted conception can wreck a woman's confidence. Some women lose their belief in their own bodies. If their bodies did not manage to conceive, why should they be able to carry a baby through to birth without constant help? This fear might be at the root of your feelings. It will mean that you will take a little time to

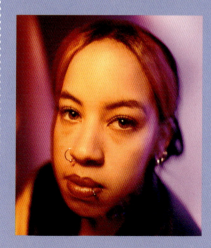

adjust to the idea that you are essentially healthy and that your body will not let you down. With each normal routine test and visit, you will gradually gain in confidence. Help your body on its way – eat a balanced diet, take exercise and practise relaxation techniques. And remember that you're not the only woman who feels this way – there are support groups (see page 106) to help you.

**Q.** I don't understand my wife. She never used to be moody before, but often now she pushes me away.

**A.** Hormones can significantly affect women in the first few months. Tiredness and fear of the unknown can then kick in later on. When your wife is moody, try hard not to take it personally and over-react. She can't help it. When she's feeling good, be close and have a laugh together. Ask yourself: Are you really listening to her? Do you show her how much you appreciate her? The occasional token of affection can go a long way in a relationship. Flowers were probably invented for this purpose.

If you have a question that isn't answered here, call Tommy's pregnancy information line on **0870 777 30 60** and speak to one of our experienced midwives.

**Q.** My partner is over seven months pregnant and I love her but our relationship is really different now. She doesn't always want to be cuddled but then she tells me that I'm not interested in her. It feels like I cannot win. I am not sure about how I feel about the baby any more.

**A.** It is not always easy to support women during their pregnancies, and at certain times some women do withdraw a little. It might be that in your relationship previously your cuddling has always gone on to mean sex. Now your partner might be avoiding cuddles because she wants affection but she is not interested in sex. Look for ways of listening to her and reassuring her that you love her. Your feelings towards the baby are being shaped by your frustration. Ask your partner if you can stroke her bump and talk to the baby. This will help your partner to see that you are interested in her and that cuddles will not necessarily lead to sex. Amazing as it seems, your baby can hear you and will learn to recognise your voice. Building this bond before the birth of the baby will help you all.

**Q.** I already have a lovely, happy daughter who is nearly two years old. I am eight months pregnant and am worrying that I may have made a big mistake. I can't see how I will be able to love the next one as much and I am frightened that my daughter will be upset and jealous.

**A.** Worrying about whether you can love another child is normal and affects fathers as well as mothers. Happily, both find that they are able to love the new baby just as easily. It's a different kind of love. Your daughter too will develop a special relationship with her new brother or sister. But she will need time to adapt to the change in the family size. Make sure she does not feel left out and once the baby has arrived, look for ways to give her some individual time. Keep finding this time, even after the first few months have gone by and everything seems settled. Older children start to react when the baby learns to crawl and become more of a presence.

**Q.** My sister had a miscarriage a few months ago and desperately wants a baby. I am finding it hard to know what to do and say when she comes around. I don't want her to be jealous because we have always been close. Our babies were due around the same time.

**A.** Many women who have had miscarriages say they find it hard when others around them have babies. It's best to be honest with each other. Tell your sister that you are struggling to find a way through this situation. She is probably finding it difficult too – while delighted for you, she is reminded of her loss, and this may make her feel guilty. Losing a baby is hard and can take a time to get over. Getting the issue out in the open will avoid misunderstandings, especially as you might still be the right person to support her. See page 106 for organisations that help support women who have lost a baby.

**top/right** Grandparents can be little bit overenthusiastic to begin with – but very helpful later on, if you tell them clearly how much you want them to be involved.

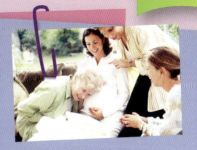

**Q.** I am five months pregnant and getting fed up with our families. Both my partner's and my own mother keep giving me advice and telling me what I should and shouldn't do. I know it will be their first grandchild, but it feels like they are trying to own the baby.

**A.** The arrival of a new baby is special in all families, but especially when it is a first grandchild. The birth of grandchildren also brings back some powerful maternal memories. This is why the prospective grandmothers are particularly enthusiastic and eager. This might be a little too much for you now, but it might be useful later, as interested grandparents can provide free babysitting and support. You might like to harness their support by finding ways to involve them in ways that do not threaten you. If they live close by, maybe they could do some of your domestic chores so that you can rest. Or nearer the time they could cook some meals for the freezer to save you time when your baby is born.

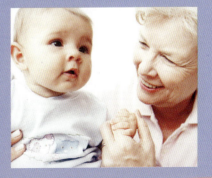

# Count down to fatherhood

Apart from a baby at the end of nine months, fathers-to-be often don't know what to expect, or what's expected of them. Here's a bit about what she's going through – and how you can help.

## The first three months (up to 13 weeks)

This is the time when much of the baby's critical development takes place. Women have a better chance of a healthy baby if they cut out smoking, avoid alcohol and drugs and take folic acid supplements. Changes in hormones also mean that women can feel incredibly tired and sick in these weeks.

### How can I help?

- Help her to rest and show her you care.
- Remember that she may need time to adjust to the idea of having a baby.
- If you both smoke, try to give up so she finds it easier to stop.
- Have plenty of alternatives to alcohol around and give her some moral support by not drinking.
- Remind her to take her folic acid supplements – 400 mcg a day for the first 12 weeks.
- Ask her if she'd like you to go with her to the doctor and booking visit.
- Make sure she seeks help immediately if she begins to bleed and be there for her if the pregnancy does end early.
- Take an interest in the changes her body is going through.

## The middle three months (Weeks 14–28)

This is a time of incredible growth. Your partner's waist will disappear, and by six months her bump will appear. She will feel the baby move and towards the end of this time, you will too. Smoking, heavy drinking and drugs will all affect your baby's health. Most women feel better in these months, and sickness has usually disappeared.

### How can I help?

- Tell her how much you care for her.
- Be ready to change your diet a little to support her. Stay away from takeaways, and go instead for healthy snacks and treats.
- Support her if she is trying to stop smoking. Every cigarette she does not smoke makes a difference to your baby's health. You can find out about quit programmes on page 106.
- Don't encourage your partner to drink by topping up her glass. An occasional drink is thought to be OK, but no more than two drinks a week. Heavy or binge drinking is definitely not advisable.
- Tell her she's beautiful – she may not feel it.
- Ask if she would like you to attend appointments with her.
- Ask her if you can attend the ultrasound scan. Show interest in the baby, by touching her bump and talking to your baby.
- Talk together about the birth.
- Organise your finances and find out about paternity leave (see page 104).

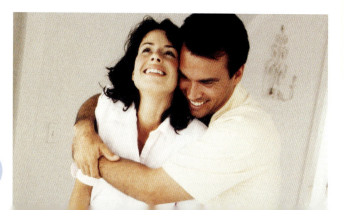

**left** Your partner will feel drained for a while and your support will make all the difference. Focus on the positive – tell her how beautiful she is, and how much you love her.

## The last three months (Weeks 29–40)

Your baby is still growing and his heart and lungs are maturing. After 28 weeks, he has a good chance of survival if he is born early. He will be able to hear you if you talk to him. Your partner may start to feel tired and heavy and worried that she won't get her shape back afterwards. She may also start to worry about giving birth.

Watch out for spring-cleaning and home improvement – many women have the instinct to get their homes ready for the baby.

## How can I help her ?

- **Encourage her to rest.**
- **Take time to be together and to focus on your baby.**
- **Show her that you care for her.**
- **Don't tease her about her size or shape!**
- **Listen to her fears about giving birth and reassure her.**
- **Help with any spring-cleaning and preparations for the baby – don't let her lift heavy stuff or go up a ladder to paint the ceiling.**
- **Plan how she can contact you if you're at work.**
- **If you are planning a hospital birth, think how you'll get her there when she's in labour.**
- **Pack a bag for yourself. Include coins, drink and snacks as well as light clothes.**
- **Talk to her about her preferences for birth (see birth plan, page 67).**
- **Read up about other methods of delivery (see page 76) so that you know what her choices are if the birth doesn't go to plan.**

## The final hurdle

No one can plan how a woman's labour will go. Some women find it easier than they'd thought, others more painful. Not all births go to plan, but there will be a team of experts on hand, which means that your baby and your partner will be in good hands.

### Stage 1

The cervix at the bottom of the womb opens ('dilates'). It needs to become 10cm dilated. This is the longest stage of the labour and for many first time mothers can be as long as 12–16 hours. In this stage most women need help to relieve the pain of the contractions. Midwives will check from time to time that the cervix is dilating. If the cervix stops dilating or it is very slow, medical intervention might be discussed.

### Stage 2

Your partner pushes your baby out of the womb. This will be quicker than the first stage – it may take around one hour – but it is very hard work. The head comes first and then the rest. The midwife checks the baby immediately. There'll be a lot of action around your partner at this stage. If your baby becomes distressed or your partner becomes too tired to push, suction, forceps or a caesarean section may be considered.

### Stage 3

The placenta is pushed out. Many men don't notice this because they're focused on their partner and the new baby. Some women may need stitches, which will be put in shortly afterwards. Soon you will enjoy having a few quiet moments alone.

## How can I help?

- **Try to stay as calm as you can.**
- **Check that she has her notes with her.**
- **If you're going to the hospital, phone ahead and don't forget your carefully pre-packed bags!**
- **Be reassuring and sensitive to her mood.**
- **Don't be surprised if she changes her mind about positions or pain relief.**
- **Stay close to your partner. Ask her if she would like you to rub her back, talk to her or hold her.**
- **Eat and drink during the first stage of labour.**
- **Don't be afraid to ask questions or make midwives aware of her needs.**
- **Encourage your partner – tell her she's doing well!**
- **Make sure that you have a camera to take some photos in the early minutes.**
- **Hold and look into the eyes of your baby.**
- **Celebrate together.**
- **Don't drive anywhere until you feel able to focus on the road!**

With all the attention focused on mum and baby, you might feel a bit left out – but this is an exciting and nervous time for you, too! Talk to your mates who are recent fathers, or save it up and talk to your partner when she's had time to recover.

# Q&A

**Q.** Will she love the baby more than me?

**A.** Mothers are generally besotted with their new babies, but this doesn't mean that you'll be pushed out. In some ways, your relationship can become stronger and deeper and she will love you more. This can only happen if you are warm, caring and supportive during the pregnancy and afterwards. You need to be part of the new package rather than be on the outside. Care for the baby and look for practical ways of helping in the next few months. Don't stand on the sidelines.

**Q.** What if I don't love the baby?

**A.** If you work hard at caring for the baby this is unlikely to be an issue. Change lots of nappies, cuddle, dress and bath your baby. The more you do for your child in the first few days and weeks, the better your relationship will be – with your child and your partner. If you want to start early, begin stroking and talking to your partner's bump.

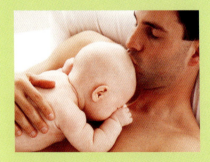

**above** Your baby will love having skin-to-skin contact with dad.

**Q.** How will I know if my partner is going into labour?

**A.** This is an important question. You might have to drop everything and leave work and get your partner to the hospital if she is not having a home birth. Some women do have a few false alarms, but most start to realise that they are properly in labour when their contractions become regular and painful. When contractions are lasting about a minute and are coming every 5–10 minutes, you should definitely be on your way. If contractions are not doing this, but your partner feels that she needs help, call your midwife, as not all labours follow the same pattern. Another sign that a woman is in labour is if her waters break. She will feel a gush of warm fluid as the amniotic fluid that has acted as a cushion for the baby in the womb starts to escape.

**Q.** How will I cope at the birth?

**A.** Most of us avoid looking at blood and seeing others in pain, so it is normal to wonder what it will be like. Happily though, birth is a bit different. You will see your child come into the world and being there will give your partner fantastic moral support. Talk to other fathers about what it is like. Most will tell you that it was one of the best moments in their lives. Be practical, too. Make sure that you pack something light to wear as well as plenty of food and water.

Bring along something to look at or do. There can be a lot of hanging around and while your partner may want you there for moral support, she may not want

you to be fussing over her. Or she may want you to be quite active and to talk and distract her. Try to take the lead from your partner and be sensitive to her mood. When it comes to the birth, most men find that they are either so busy supporting their partner women or so excited by the birth, that the blood doesn't seem quite so important.

**Q.** What about sex?

**A.** Sex is fine during pregnancy, as long as your partner feels like it and the doctor has not said otherwise. How often and when your partner feels like sex will vary during the pregnancy. In some weeks your partner may be really keen, but don't be surprised if in others she is not interested at all. Try to go with the flow and not force the issue. Your partner needs you to be understanding rather than demanding. Get into the habit of cuddling and hugging your partner without expecting sex. She will love you for this, and this will bring you closer together.

After your partner has given birth, you need to follow the doctor's guidelines. In general, this means waiting until your partner feels ready. She might be feeling exhausted and nervous. Plan ahead, buy some lubricant and be ready to let her set the pace. Be ready to stop if things get too uncomfortable, especially if your partner has had any stitches. Don't worry if it doesn't go very well. Failed erections, leaky breasts and crying babies are all normal. Try to have a laugh and a cuddle. Working on the relationship will help you both to relax and make love again when the time is right.

# Just like the movies

When Neil's partner Karen went into labour his car was blocked in. Neil shouted that Karen was having a baby and the driver moved off sharpish! Here Neil, 28, gives his own account of becoming a dad – from the first news to the day he held baby Euan in his arms for the first time.

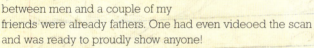

Karen phoned me at work to tell me she was pregnant. It stopped me in my tracks as, although we had been trying, I wasn't really expecting it. You always wonder as a man whether or not you are able to do it and so to be honest it was a bit of a relief. It can be quite competitive out there between men and a couple of my friends were already fathers. One had even videoed the scan and was ready to proudly show anyone!

During the pregnancy, I think that it took time to get used to the idea that we were going to be three. Going to the scan was really important, though. I wanted to be a part of it and I wanted to support Karen. I realised quite early on in the pregnancy, that once a man has done his bit, he has to take second place. At the scan, Karen was the focus of the attention and although the sonographer did talk to me, quite a lot is aimed at the woman. That didn't bother me because I knew that Karen needed me there. I was just pleased to see the heart move and to find out that all was well. I attended some of the antenatal classes too. While that kind of thing is not normally what I would choose to do, it was useful and I did get the idea of what would be happening during the birth.

A month before the baby was due, I was made redundant. That was really hard because when you know there is a baby on the way, you want to be able to provide for it. I did get another job quickly, but it was stressful. It was hard too because I didn't want to tell Karen about my worries. I think that as a man, you sometimes just have to get on with it. I also wondered about whether I'd be able to cope watching her in labour. Thoughts also went through my head about what would happen if the baby was stillborn or had a problem. Again, it's not something that you can tell others about and I had to keep pushing these thoughts away. I knew that

Karen wanted me to be there and although I didn't know how it would go or what I would feel, I knew that I just had to be there because that's what she wanted.

The due date came and went. I knew that babies did not always arrive on time, but I had in my mind set myself the date. When Karen did go into labour, she was quite calm. When we got to the car, I couldn't get out straight away as another car was blocking the way. After a few moments, I got out and shouted at the driver that my wife was having a baby. That made them move and it was just like the line from a film!

In the delivery room, I just followed Karen's mood and looked for ways of helping. She had gas and air and needed sips of water in between because her mouth became dry. The midwife would pop in and out and it was strange being there together when we were on our own. I felt quite responsible and was pleased that I was with her. The time goes very quickly and you can forget to eat and drink yourself. When the time comes to push, things really get moving. I listened carefully to what the midwife was saying and made sure that I wasn't in the way.

I tried deliberately not to look down there, but when the head was coming through, I did have a look. I remember thinking that this was a once in a lifetime moment and it would be stupid to miss it. The excitement of seeing your baby born means that you don't really notice what else is happening. I also saw Karen in a new light. I really admired how she coped and the whole birth made us much closer together. I had hoped that I might be able to cut the cord, but Euan needed to be helped to breathe and so the midwife whipped him away.

I am pleased that I was there. Not only for Karen, but also for myself. It sounds silly, but I was proud that I had gone through it too and been a part of it. I love being a dad and it does change your life. You can see why other dads are proud and once you have a child, you wouldn't go back. At least I wouldn't.

" *The whole birth made us much closer* "

# More than one baby – twins and multiples

Finding out that you are having more than one baby can come as a surprise. We look at what this might mean for you and your pregnancy.

## Finding out

Most multiple pregnancies are confirmed with a scan. Twins and multiple births are also more common after fertility treatment.

## Extra care for you

If you are expecting more than one baby, your healthcare team will take extra care of you and your pregnancy. You may be offered additional antenatal appointments and scans. You are also likely to be advised to rest – especially during the last few months – to give your body a chance to cope and to avoid going into labour early. You may find that you need this extra rest as a multiple pregnancy can be more tiring. Women often find that they get more than their fair share of minor problems such as backache, sleeplessness and indigestion.

A multiple pregnancy is not always easy. To spot and deal with potential complications, your antenatal team will want to keep a close eye on you and it is likely, for example, that you will be advised to have your babies in hospital. A caesarean is also an option that your obstetrician is likely to discuss with you, though it is not always needed. Around half of women carrying twins are delivered vaginally – it depends how well you are, the position of the babies and what happens in labour.

## Special care for your babies

Some multiple pregnancies go on for the full term, sometimes the babies arrive early. Pregnancy complications are more common in multiple births and an obstetrician may advise that the babies are safer delivered early, this can mean that they need to have extra care and go into a special care baby unit (SCBU – see page 81).

## Mixed reactions

If you've been expecting one baby, finding out there's more than one feels like going on a rollercoaster ride. Most women and their partners admit to feeling shocked and concerned about how they'll cope. As the pregnancy continues, most people find that they gradually adjust and are able to start thinking how they'll manage looking after more than one baby. Support groups like the Twins and Multiple Births Association (TAMBA) (address on page 106) offer practical advice and emotional support.

## Feeding your babies

You can breastfeed your babies, which will get them off to a flying start. Some women feed twins together, one on each breast, while others take one baby at a time. It's also possible to express your milk to give in a bottle, so that your partner can help with feeding. Your midwife and local TAMBA group can support you with breastfeeding.

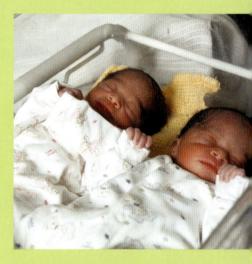

**above** There is plenty of support if you are expecting twins or more.

## Practical help

Think ahead about how you'll care for more than one. Your partner can take paid paternity leave and other family members and friends may help you. Try contacting local colleges that offer childcare qualifications. They may be able to provide you with a trainee student. You can also contact Home-Start who offer volunteer support to parents of young children (details on page 106). You might also like to find out about organisations in your area that help new mums. Home-Start (see page 106) has trained volunteers to help with pre-school age children. It can also be worth contacting social services to see if they can offer any support.

# Your rights & benefits

There are many rights and benefits that it is worth knowing about when you are pregnant. Here's what you might be able to claim and how you can find out more.

## Get moving!

It may seem a long time till you give birth, but you must think about claiming benefits and asking for maternity leave as soon as you can. If you put it off you can lose out financially. Your right to benefits and time off work does not come automatically. You have to claim them. There are plenty of places you can go to find out more, and get help with filling in forms. These include

- **Social security office**
- **JobCentre Plus**
- **Department of Work and Pensions**
- **Maternity Alliance**
- **Citizen's Advice Bureau**
- **Inland Revenue**

There are details of helplines and websites for these organisations on page 106.

## The must haves!

### Free prescriptions form (FW8)

You're entitled to free prescriptions and dental care while you're pregnant and for a year after your baby is born. Once your pregnancy is confirmed, ask your doctor or midwife for the form FW8 and send it off to your Health Authority, who will send you an exemption card.

## Maternity Certificate (MAT B1)

When you are 20 weeks pregnant you need to get a maternity certificate MAT B1 from your midwife or doctor. This certificate is important to get maternity leave and benefits. Give this to your employer.

## Child Benefit claim pack

Child benefit is a weekly payment for each child. Everyone with children is eligible, but you need to claim it. You can get the form now so that you have it available for later. Ask or phone your local Inland Revenue office for a Child Benefit claim pack or download the details from the Inland Revenue website (see page 106).

## Child Tax Credit

If you or your partner works, ask for a Child Tax Credit pack from the Inland Revenue after your baby is born. The amount of income tax you pay on your wages might then be reduced.

## Time off work

### Attending clinics, doctor's appointments and classes

You are entitled to reasonable time off work so that you can see your doctor, attend clinics and go to your antenatal classes. This is paid time off work, so you will not lose out financially. Keep on good terms with your employer by letting them know in advance when you need the time off. Your employer can

ask to see your appointment card or a certificate stating you are pregnant.

## Maternity leave

You will need some time off work to have your baby. You will also need some time off before and after the birth. You have the right to maternity leave and more importantly to return to the same job afterwards. There are two types of maternity leave: Ordinary Maternity Leave and Additional Maternity Leave.

**below** Ask your midwife if you need help filling in the forms.

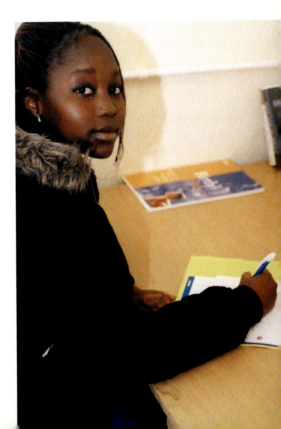

| Type of leave | Can I get it? | How long is it? | What do I do? | Will I get anything? |
|---|---|---|---|---|
| **Ordinary Maternity Leave (OML)** | For all employed women even if you have only been working for your employer for a few days. | Total of 26 weeks from the day you start your maternity leave. You can decide how to use the leave before and after the birth, but you cannot start maternity leave until 11 weeks before the baby is due. For example, you could take 11 weeks before and 15 weeks after, or three weeks before and 23 weeks after. | You must write to your employer at least 28 days before you intend to take the maternity leave and claim Statutory Maternity Pay. | You may be able to get Statutory Maternity Pay (SMP) or Maternity Allowance. |
| **Additional Maternity Leave** | You must have worked for your employer for at least 26 weeks by the 15th week before your baby is due. | This follows on from your Ordinary Maternity leave and lasts for 26 weeks. | If you are eligible for it, you don't need to tell your employer if you want to add AML to Ordinary Maternity Leave. | You may be able to get Statutory Maternity Pay (SMP) or Maternity Allowance for the first 18 weeks of your leave. |
| **Statutory Paternity Leave (for prospective dads!)** | You must have worked for this employer for at least nine months by the time the baby is due. You must be earning enough to be paying National Insurance. | Up to two weeks in one block. This leave must be taken by the eighth week after the baby's birth, or due date if the baby is born early. | Tell your employer when you intend to take leave by the 15th week before the baby is due | You will get a fixed allowance of £102.80 a week (2004 rates) or 90% of your average weekly pay, whichever is the smaller. |

## Getting paid while you are on maternity leave

Whether you're paid while on maternity leave depends on:
- How long you have worked for your employer.
- How much you are paid.
- How much National Insurance you have paid.

## Statutory Maternity Pay (SMP)

Your employer pays this allowance for the 26 weeks when you take maternity leave. It doesn't matter if you intend to return to work or not. You should check with your employer that you qualify, but as a rough guide you need to:
- Have been working for at least six months for the same employer before you became pregnant
- Still be in work 15 weeks before the baby is due
- Earn enough to pay National Insurance contributions
- Have left work to take maternity leave or because your job was made redundant.

**To claim SMP**, you need to write to your employer and tell them when you intend to start maternity leave and ask them to pay you SMP. You will need to give them a copy of your maternity certificate MAT B1.

**For the first six weeks,** you will get 90% of your average weekly pay. **For the next twenty weeks**, you will get a flat-rate allowance.

## Maternity Allowance

This is paid for women who do not qualify for Statutory Maternity Pay. You might be able to claim this allowance if:
- You have changed jobs during pregnancy.
- You are self-employed.
- You have had low earnings or have been unemployed during your pregnancy.

To claim Maternity Allowance, you need form MA1, which you can get from your local benefits agency or antenatal clinic or download from the internet (see page 106). You can fill in this form once you are 26 weeks pregnant. You will also need to send your maternity certificate MAT B1. If you are employed you will need a form SMP1 from your employer which explains why you cannot claim the higher SMP.

## Not in work or on a low income?

There are other benefits for women who are not working or who are on a low income. The best way of finding out about these is to visit your benefits office or go to your Citizen's Advice Bureau.

## SureStart Maternity Grant

If you are on a low income and receiving benefits, find out whether you can claim the SureStart Maternity Grant (see page 106). You can use this lump sum of money to buy baby equipment and clothes. You do not have to pay this back.

# True or false?

There are many myths around pregnancy and birth. See if you can spot the facts from the fiction!

## A pregnant woman needs to eat for two

**False.** You need to eat a balanced diet with plenty of fruit and vegetables, but you do not have to eat for two. Eating too many fatty and sugary foods will simply mean that you put on excess weight.

## If you smoke during pregnancy, you will have an easier birth

**False.** Smoking harms your own health and gives your baby a poor start. Babies of smokers tend to be lighter, but this does not mean an easier birth. There is also a significant risk of babies being born prematurely, which can affect their ability to survive. If you do smoke, try to give up or, if this is impossible, cut down as much as you possibly can. Your midwife can help you find a quit smoking programme or find details on page 106.

## Sex can be better during pregnancy and will do no harm

**True.** Many women find that sex gets better in pregnancy once they are past the first few weeks. This is due to the extra supply of blood and sensation to the vagina. Sex will not do any harm to the baby except in very rare cases.

## Scratching during late pregnancy is a sign that you will have a boy

**False**. The only ways to tell the sex of a baby are during an ultrasound scan or from an amniocentesis or chorionic villus sampling test (see page 39). While mild itching is common in middle and late pregnancy, severe itching, especially on the hands and feet, can be a sign of a liver disorder called obstetric cholestasis and so is always worth mentioning to your midwife.

**Say again?** Obstetric cholestasis is a rare condition of pregnancy that affects the liver. It can put both mother and baby at risk. The symptoms are severe itching, and you should not ignore them. Tell your doctor or midwife straightaway.

## You can still get pregnant when you are breastfeeding

**True.** Breastfeeding can reduce a woman's fertility, but it is not a good idea to rely on it as a contraceptive. If you do not want another baby straightaway, you will need to use contraception.

## Bottlefeeding is easier than breastfeeding

**False.** When it comes to convenience as well as a head start for your baby, breastfeeding wins every time. Bottlefeeding means sterilising bottles, heating them up and waiting for them to cool down while your baby is crying. Breastfeeding means that your milk is permanently on tap!

## A caesarean is better because of your sex life afterwards

**False.** The vagina does stretch to allow you to give birth, but it then shrinks to its previous size, making no difference to your sex life. Any tears soon heal. Caesarean sections are major operations and should be seen as a last rather than a first resort.

## Most babies do not arrive on time

**True.** Only one baby in 30 is born on their due date. Most babies are born within a week either side of their due date whether they are the first, second or ninth baby!

## You should avoid exercising during pregnancy

**False.** It is important to rest during pregnancy, but this is not an excuse to become a couch potato. Regular gentle exercise will tone your body, strengthen your muscles, and help you to get back into shape earlier.

## You should not have baths when you are pregnant

**False.** You can have baths during pregnancy as they are quite relaxing and will not harm the baby. Be sensible about the temperature of the water as very hot water is not good for you. Ideally you should be able to sit comfortably in the water and take your time.

# signposts

The following organisations can give you further information about the topics covered in this book. They're grouped into sections to help you find the best one for you.

## Pregnancy and birth

### Tommy's, the baby charity
Nicholas House
3 Laurence Pountney Hill
London EC4R 0BB
*Pregnancy information line:*
0870 777 30 60
www.tommys.org

Tommy's provides information for parents, parents-to-be, health professionals and the general public, to help maximise the chance of having a healthy pregnancy, through a telephone pregnancy information line, email and web access to health professionals, plus a range of free publications. Tommy's also funds a national programme of medical research and information

### NHS Direct
0845 4647
www.nhsdirect.nhs.uk
A 24-hour nurse advice and health information service

### Birth Choice UK
www.birthchoiceuk.com
A clickable online map that compares maternity units in your area

### Independent Midwives Association
01483 821104
www.independentmidwives.org.uk
Register of accredited independent midwives

### Active Birth Centre
020 7281 6760
www.activebirthcentre.com
Support and information if you want to give birth as naturally as possible

### National Childbirth Trust
0870 444 8707
www.nctpregnancyandbabycare.com
Antenatal classes, postnatal and breastfeeding support

### Women's Health Information Centre
www.womenshealthlondon.org.uk
*Helpline* 0845 125 5254 *(Mon to Fri 9.30am–1.30pm)*
Provides health information and advice on a wide range of women's health issues including contraception

## Pregnancy testing and contraception

### British Pregnancy Advisory Service
08457 30 40 30
www.bpas.org
Confidential counselling and information service for women feeling unsure about their pregnancy

### fpa (formerly Family Planning Association)
*England and Wales* 0845 310 1334
*Scotland* 0141 576 5088
*Northern Ireland* 028 90 325 488
www.fpa.org.uk
Confidential advice service on sexual health and reproductive issues

### Brook
0800 0185 023
www.brook.org.uk
Confidential advice service on sexual health for young people

### Antenatal Results and Choices
020 7631 0285
www.arc-uk.org
Offers support for parents throughout the antenatal testing process and when abnormalities are diagnosed

## Complementary therapies
For a list of accredited practitioners in your area:

### Association for Professional Hypnosis and Psychotherapy
01702 347691
www.aphp.net

### British Osteopathic Association
01582 488455
www.findanosteopath.co.uk

### British Acupuncture Council
020 8735 0400
www.acupuncture.org.uk

### National Institute of Medical Herbalists
01932 426022
www.nimh.org.uk
*Herbal Advice Line* 0906 8020177 *(calls cost 60p/min) Mon to Fri 9am to 1pm*
Advice on how to take herbal remedies, interaction of herbs with other medication and safe use of herbs for children and during pregnancy

## Rights and benefits

### Maternity Alliance
020 7490 7628
www.maternityalliance.org.uk
Information and legal advice on aspects of maternity benefits and rights with detailed fact-sheets available on rights for pregnant women

### Citizens Advice Bureau
www.adviceguide.org.uk
www.citizensadvice.org.uk *(for a list of centres closest to you)*
Provides advice to help people resolve their debt, benefits, housing, legal, discrimination, employment, immigration,

consumer and other problems; advisors can help fill out forms, and explain benefits and available assistance

## Tax credits
0845 300 3900
www.taxcredits.inlandrevenue.gov.uk
Information on tax credits such as Working Tax Credit and Children's Tax Credit

## Child benefit Office
0845 302 1444
www.inlandrevenue.gov.uk/childbenefit
Provides information about eligibility for child benefit, with forms available online

## TIGER (Tailored Interactive Guidance on Employment Rights)
www.tiger.gov.uk
User-friendly website about employment rights, includes an interactive calculator to help parents and employers work out leave and pay entitlements, and a calendar to help women plan their maternity leave

## Jobcentre plus
www.jobcentreplus.gov.uk
A general guide to eligibility for benefits

## Help with a new baby

### Children's information services
0800 096 02 96
www.childcarelink.gov.uk
Face-to-face or phone advice on all aspects of childcare, and details of childcare in your local area

### Sure Start
www.surestart.gov.uk
Sure Start is the Government's programme to deliver the best start in life for every child by bringing together: early education, childcare, health and family support

### Home-Start
08000 68 63 68
www.home-start.org.uk
Home-Start offers support and practical help to parents with young children in local communities throughout the UK; volunteers are usually parents themselves and can visit families at home

## Help to quit or cut down

### QUIT
0800 00 22 00
www.quit.org.uk
Email and text message support to give up smoking

### National Drugs Helpline
0800 77 66 00
www.talktofrank.com
Advice and information on services and support available for drug-related problems

### NHS Pregnancy smoking helpline
0800 169 9 169
www.givingupsmoking.co.uk
Support, advice and information for women trying to get pregnant or currently pregnant about stopping smoking

### Drinkline
0800 917 8282
www.wrecked.co.uk
Support and information about alcohol related concerns

## Special pregnancies

### APEC
(Action on pre-eclampsia)
020 8427 4217
www.apec.org.uk
Support and information about this life-threatening condition of pregnancy

### Obstetric Cholestasis Trust
0121 353 0699
Information line for women who have suffered from this dangerous condition of pregnancy or who think they may have it

### Hyperemesis Gravidarum Awareness Group (Blooming Awful)
07050 655 094
Email: support@hyperemesis.org.uk
(preferable to phone enquiries)
www.hyperemesis.org.uk
Support group run by volunteers for women suffering severe sickness and nausea throughout entire pregnancy

### Ectopic Pregnancy Trust
01895 238 025
www.ectopic.org.uk
Support and information for women and their families whose lives have been affected by an ectopic pregnancy

## GBSS (Group B Strep support)
01444 410 170 (manned intermittently/ answerphone)
Information and support for women and their families whose lives have been affected by an ectopic pregnancy

## TAMBA
(Twins and Multiple Birth Association)
Twins and multiple birth association (tamba)
01732 868000
www.tamba.org.uk
Support and information for families with twins or more

## ACE babes
www.acebabes.co.uk
'Bump buddies' – support for parents-to-be who have had IVF or other assisted conception

## When a baby dies

### SANDS
(Stillbirth and Neonatal Death Society)
020 7436 5881
www.uk-sands.org
Support and information for bereaved parents and their families when their baby dies at or soon after birth, with support for next pregnancy

### Miscarriage Association
England and Wales  01924 200 799
Scotland  0131 334 8883
www.miscarriageassociation.org.uk
Support and information for women who have miscarried; and their partners, and families; with support for next pregnancy

## Websites
Many websites offer useful information for your pregnancy, breastfeeding, childcare and more. For online magazines, message boards and due date calculators you can start with these:

**Babyworld:** www.babyworld.co.uk
**BabyCentre:** www.babycentre.co.uk
**Bounty:** www.bounty.com
**BBC Parenting:** www.bbc.co.uk/parenting

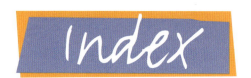

# Index

abbreviations 24–25, 37
abortion previously 14, 30
addresses, useful 106
air travel 35, 56, 71, 84
alcohol 15, 88
allergies 87
amniotic fluid 36
    amniocentesis 39, 42
    amniotomy 76
anaemia 40, 88, 95
anaesthetic 65–66
    local or regional 76, 80
antenatal
    care 18–22, 24–25, 58–59
    classes 19, 43–45
anus 27
appointments 19, 30, 38, 58
    booking visit 20–21
areola 26
aromatherapy 64, 89
augmentation [by drip] 76

baby in womb (fetus) 19, 25, 60
    at 1–12 weeks 10–11, 26
    at 13–28 weeks 32–35
    at 29–40 weeks 27, 54–56
baby (newborn) 78–79
    clothes and equipment 50, 54,
        69, 70
    overdue 82
    premature 54, 56, 81
backache 46, 93
baths, warm 64, 105
belly ring [body piercing] 52
birth canal 27
birth plan 67–68, 71, 72
bladder 26
    leaking 47, 56, 79, 94
bleeding 29, 79
    light (spotting) 6, 10, 29, 35
blood 21, 40, 79
    sugar 16, 21
    pressure 21, 95
body parts (organs) 26–27
booking visit 20–21
boyfriend see partner and
    fatherhood
bra, support 11, 12, 34, 69
breastfeeding 50, 78, 105
breasts 6, 12, 26, 56
    leaking 34, 46, 69
breech position 59, 72, 80

caesarean section 80, 105
carpal tunnel syndrome 62, 94
cats and toxoplasmosis 31, 87
cervical smear test 21
cervix 27, 72
children 20, 97
chorionic villus sampling (CVS)
    39
clitoris 27
clubbing (going out) 15
clumsiness 56
colostrum 34, 46
complementary medicine 45,
    64, 89
conception difficulties 96
constipation 12, 47, 93
contact lenses 55
contraceptives 10, 31
contractions 72–73, 75

Braxton Hicks 56, 62
cramp [pain] 29, 37, 79, 94
CTG (cardiotocograph) 75

deep vein thrombosis 37
dentist 34
diaphragm 26
doctor (GP) 9, 18, 22, 35, 49
    finding another 19
domino scheme 19
doula [companion] 63
Down's syndrome 39, 40, 42
dreams 62
drinks 16, 69, 85, 88, 94
    alcohol 15, 88
    caffeine 87
    raspberry leaf tea 82
    water 16, 35, 56, 88, 92
drip [giving drug] 76
drugs 89
    recreational 19, 30, 89
due date 8, 9, 105

eating 16, 47, 69, 82, 84–87, 88
ectopic pregnancies 28
ECV (external cephalic version)
    59
EDD (estimated due date) 8
embryo [baby in womb] 25
employer see work
engaging (baby moving head-
    down) 56
Entonox (gas & air) [pain relief]
    65, 66
epidural [pain relief] 65, 66
episiotomy [operation] 76
ERPC (operation) 29
exercise 15, 62, 91–92, 105
    breathing 64
    pelvic floor 9
eyes, baby's 36, 55
eyesight 52

faintness 7, 13, 93
father see partner and
    fatherhood
fatty acids, essential 84
FBS (fetal blood sampling) 75
feelings 7, 10–11, 14, 31, 32–35,
    54–56, 96–97
fetus see baby in womb
finger pains 62, 94
fluids see drinks
folic acid 10, 84
fontanelles 78
food 16, 47, 69, 82, 84–87, 88
forceps 76
forms 34, 103–104
FSE (fetal scalp electrode) 75
full term 10
fundus (top of womb) 25

German measles (rubella) 40
going out (clubbing) 15
GP see doctor
grandparents 97
Group B streptococcus 95

haemoglobin (Hb) 24
haemorrhoids (piles) 47, 93
hair dye 36
HCG [hormone] 8, 37
headaches 12, 52, 58
health visitor 22
healthy tips 10–11, 32–35,
    54–56
heartbeat 11
    baby's 33
heartburn 47, 93
hepatitis B 40, 79
herbal remedies 89
HIV and AIDS 40
holiday 35, 56, 71, 84
home birth 49, 51
home, going home from
    hospital 79
homeopathy 64
hormones 7, 37
hospital birth 44, 45, 49
husband see partner and
    fatherhood
hygiene 87
hypnosis, self- 64

illnesses you already have 95
internal examination (VE) 21, 82
interventions 76
iron tablets 88
itchiness 62
IVF (in vitro fertilisation) 96

labour 72–76
lanugo [hair] 34
lifting things 56, 91, 92
lightening [when baby
    engages] 56
linea nigra (black line) 11
Listeria [bacterium] 87

maternity leave 55
medication 88, 89, 95
membrane sweep 82
midwife 19, 20, 22–23, 30, 49,
    74, 77, 79
miscarriage 14, 28–29, 97
morning sickness 7, 12, 16–17,
    93
movement in womb 29, 36

nausea (feeling sick) 7, 12
negative test results 30
nipples 26, 82
nosebleeds 78
notes, your 21, 24–25, 72
nuchal translucency scan 39
nutrients 36

obstetric cholestasis 105
obstetrician 22, 57
oedema (swelling) 25, 47, 79,
    94
oestrogen [hormone] 37
ovaries 27, 33
overdue babies 82
oxytocin [hormone] 72
oxytocinons [drugs] 76

packing and what to pack 69
pains and symptoms 20, 93–95
    pain relief 63–66
palpation 38
partner and fatherhood 9, 21,
    31, 52, 98–100
    at the birth 50, 100–101
    how he can help 71, 83, 98–99
    how he feels 96–97, 100
    sex while pregnant 13, 97,
        100
    uninterested 15, 20, 97
pee see urine (wee)
pelvis 27, 61
perineum 27, 76
periods (menstruation) 6
pessary 82
Pethidine [pain relief] 65, 66
photographs 53, 69, 99
physical problems 12–14, 20,
    46–48, 61–62, 93–95
piles (haemorrhoids) 47, 93
pill (contraceptive) 31
placenta 33, 36, 37, 56, 75, 81
    praevia (low-lying) 59, 80
poo (baby's excrement) 78–79
positions 75
    of baby 59, 72, 80
positive test results 30, 39
postnatal care 79
pre-eclampsia (PET) 25, 40, 58,
    81
pregnancy tests 8, 30
premature babies 54, 56, 81
primigravida 25
problems 12–14, 20, 46–48,
    61–62, 93–95
progesterone [hormone] 37
prostaglandin [drug] 82
pubic hair 27
puffiness (swelling) 25, 47, 79,
    94

questions & answers 20, 59
    Am I pregnant? 6–8, 30
    Am I really having a
        miscarriage? 28–29
    Am I starting labour? 72–73,
        83

raspberry leaf tea 82
rectum 26
reflexology 64
rib pain 61
rights and benefits 103–104

Salmonella [bacterium] 87
scans 21, 41, 51, 52
SCBU (Special Care Baby Unit)
    81
scratching 105
screening see tests
sex of the baby 52
sex while pregnant 13, 82, 97,
    100, 105
show [spots of blood] 61, 62, 72
sick see morning sickness;
    nausea
sickle-cell anaemia 40, 42, 79
sleep 56, 61, 71, 83
smells 17
    smelly discharge 34, 62, 79

smoking 15, 89, 90, 105
sonographer (radiographer) 41
spina bifida 40, 42
spotting [light bleeding] 6, 10,
    29, 35
stay in hospital 79, 80, 81
streptococcus Group B 95
stress 48
stretch marks 53
sweating 34, 79
swelling (oedema) 25, 47, 79,
    94
syntocinon [drug] 76, 82
syntometrine [drug] 76
syphilis 40

tampons 29, 62, 69
teeth and gums 34, 47, 94
temperature, high 35, 47, 79
TENS [pain relief] 64
tests 21, 39–41, 51
    baby 79
    pregnancy 8, 30
thalassaemia 40, 79
thrush [infection] 48, 94
thyroid [gland] 79
Tommy's midwife 18
toxoplasmosis 31, 87
trimesters [3-month terms] 10
triple test 39
true or false? 105
tummy [abdomen] 38
    ache or pain 12, 61
twins 35, 81, 102

ultrasound see scans
urine (wee) 16
    leaking 47, 56, 79, 94
    sample 21
    weeing constantly 6, 12, 94
uterus (womb) 26, 27

vagina 21, 27
    discharge 34, 56, 62, 79
    examination (VE) 21, 82
varicose veins 48, 93
VBAC (vaginal birth after
    caesarean) 80
veins 26, 37
ventouse [suction pad] 76
vernix [coating] 78
vitamin K 79
vomiting 16, 58, 95
vulva 27

water birth 50, 67
waters breaking 29, 56, 73–74,
    76
wee see urine
week-by-week guide 10–11,
    32–35, 54–56
weight gain 13, 53, 86
    baby's 27, 56, 79
weight loss 16, 88
where to have my baby 49
wind (flatulence) 13
womb see uterus
work 33, 48
    and benefits 21, 55, 103–104
    time off 31, 44, 52, 55

X-rays 11